IMPROVING OUTCOMES IN CHRONIC HEART FAILURE:
A practical guide to specialist nurse intervention

Edited by

SIMON STEWART
Honorary Research Fellow/National Heart Foundation of Australia
Post-Doctoral Overseas Research Fellow,
University of Glasgow,
United Kingdom

and

LYNDA BLUE
Nurse Coordinator,
Greater Glasgow Primary Care NHS Trust,
Glasgow, United Kingdom

First published in 2001
by BMJ Books, BMA House, Tavistock Square,
London WC1H 9JR

www.bmjbooks.com

British Library Cataloguing in Publication Data

A catalogue record for this book is available from the British Library

ISBN 0-7279-1591-6

Typeset by FiSH Books, London
Printed and bound by MPG Books, Bodmin, Cornwall

Contents

Contributors

Lynda Blue
Nurse Coordinator
Heart Failure Nurse Service
Greater Glasgow Primary Care NHS Trust
Glasgow
United Kingdom

Charles Cline
Consultant Cardiologist
Department of Cardiology
Malmö University Hospital
Lund University
S-205 02 Malmö
Sweden

Robert N Doughty
New Zealand National Heart Foundation BNZ Senior Fellow
Department of Medicine
Faculty of Medicine and Health Science
The University of Auckland
New Zealand

Kathleen Dracup
Dean, School of Nursing
University of California in San Francisco
USA

John D Horowitz
Professor, Department of Cardiology
The Queen Elizabeth Hospital/University of Adelaide
Woodville
Australia

Anneli Iwarson
Research Nurse
Department of Cardiology
Malmö University Hospital
Lund University
S-205 02 Malmö
Sweden

Tiny Jaarsma
Scientific Advisor on Heart Failure
Netherlands Heart Foundation
PO Box 300
2501 CH, The Hague,
The Netherlands

Karen H Martens
Professor
Capital University
Columbus, Ohio
USA

John JV McMurray
Professor, Clinical Research Initiative in Heart Failure
Wolfson Building
University of Glasgow
United Kingdom

Stephanie Muncaster
Research Nurse, Department of Medicine
Faculty of Medicine and Health Science
The University of Auckland
New Zealand

Ann Pearl
Research Fellow, Department of Medicine
Faculty of Medicine and Health Science
The University of Auckland
New Zealand

Norman Sharpe
Professor, Department of Medicine
Faculty of Medicine and Health Science
The University of Auckland
New Zealand

Simon Stewart
Honorary Research Fellow/National Heart Foundation of Australia
Post-Doctoral Overseas Research Fellow
MRC Clinical Research Initiative in Heart Failure
Wolfson Building
University of Glasgow
United Kingdom

Helen J Walsh
Research Nurse
Research Fellow, Department of Medicine
Faculty of Medicine and Health Science
The University of Auckland
New Zealand

Sue P Wright
Research Fellow, Department of Medicine
Faculty of Medicine and Health Science
The University of Auckland
New Zealand

Foreword

Heart failure constitutes a major health problem and is quickly becoming a worldwide epidemic. It is a leading cause of morbidity and mortality in industrialised countries and, increasingly, in developing countries. As the incidence and prevalence of heart failure increases around the world, healthcare professionals are beginning to look beyond the development of new drugs and surgical procedures and focus on the systems of care in which patients are diagnosed and treated. In fact, many clinicians have come to realise that the best, most cutting edge treatments are ineffective if the system in which the patient is treated does not promote patient self management and the involvement of the family and other support systems. A modern silver bullet delivered in an archaic wheel barrow will never hit the target effectively. Given the high costs of caring for patients with heart failure, it is essential that we systematically test the manner in which care is provided, just as we test the treatment modalities themselves.

This textbook is unique from several perspectives. First, it is the first textbook on heart failure to offer an international perspective. Dr Stewart and Ms Blue have gathered experts from many countries to consider the issues surrounding the care of patients with heart failure. Because they come from a variety of cultures and healthcare systems, these authors are able to pose innovative and creative approaches to respond to the many challenges involved in caring for patients with heart failure.

Second, the book goes far beyond the usual consideration of diagnosis and treatment. It focuses on the way to organise the care the patient receives. Nurses who are developing heart failure programs where none have existed before face many challenges in trying to organise a different structure of patient care. The authors address the many practical aspects of starting a program. Many healthcare organisations are considering how to best create a systematic way to address the errors of diagnosis and treatment that frequently occur in this population and result in frequent rehospitalisations. Administrators and/or physicians ask nurses to mount a heart failure program, but until the publication of this textbook there has been no way for nurses to get the information they need to start such a program.

Third, the contributors represent the interdisciplinary collaboration that is the hallmark of effective care in this patient population. Physicians working predominately in the out-patient setting with many constraints on their time have found patients with heart failure a challenging target of care. Teaching patients to become knowledgeable partners in their own care requires an extraordinary amount of time. The organisation of heart failure programs that promote effective collaboration of nurses, physicians and other professionals (e.g., dieticians, social workers pharmacists) is the only way to make heart failure programs cost-effective in the long run. In many of the chapters you will find interdisciplinary collaboration a critical part of the presentation.

Finally, this book allows the reader access to some of the world authorities on heart failure programs. Publishing constraints by journals make it impossible to give all the data that experts would like to share with other healthcare professionals. This book has given many of them the forum that they have needed to explain their experiences and the dynamics behind the data reported in various journal articles. It is a fascinating read.

Kathleen Dracup
Dean and Professor
School of Nursing
University of California, San Francisco, USA

Preface

Heart failure is rapidly becoming the most important chronic cardiac condition in developed countries. Despite the development and introduction of more effective pharmacological agents in the treatment of this complex syndrome, heart failure continues to be associated with frequent hospitalisation, poor quality of life and premature mortality.

The typical complexity of managing individuals with heart failure who have been discharged from acute hospital care requires an equally complex but flexible response to ensure better health outcomes. In recent years it has been increasingly recognised that specialist nurse-led programmes have the potential to significantly improve health outcomes in heart failure through the co-ordination of more individualised and considerate care. However, putting research into practice is always difficult, especially when the only available information comes from abbreviated study reports in peer-reviewed journals.

It is within this context that we have brought together an international panel of nursing and medical experts who have been instrumental in developing and introducing this type of intervention. These experts provide detailed reports of their interventions and discuss the implications of their own and their international counterparts' research. Based on the combined wisdom of these experts and our own experience in introducing a specialist nurse-led service in a major metropolitan centre in the United Kingdom, we have provided a detailed description of how best to develop and introduce a successful service of this type.

Simon Stewart
Lynda Blue

1: The increasing burden of chronic heart failure

JOHN JV McMURRAY, SIMON STEWART

Introduction

Although cardiovascular mortality rates have declined appreciably in most industrialised countries since the 1970s, coronary heart disease continues to be a major contributor to morbidity and mortality in Western society.[1] Although impressive inroads have been made into the incidence of coronary heart disease in the past few decades, the trend towards larger and significantly older populations in developed countries[2] and better overall treatment of coronary heart disease among younger individuals has meant that its prevalence has increased markedly in older people.[1]

A major advance in confronting the impact of heart disease has been the significant reduction in the number of "premature deaths", the result of more effective primary prevention, acute treatment, and secondary prevention strategies, which reduce the risk of developing coronary heart disease, improve the immediate prognosis for individuals who do experience an acute coronary event, and improve their subsequent prognostic outlook.

Paradoxically, however, the initially improved survival prospects of individuals with acute myocardial infarction (for example) have no doubt contributed to an older patient population more susceptible to morbidity associated with advanced coronary heart disease and in particular the development of chronic heart failure.[1] The problems associated with a greater prevalence of older individuals with coronary heart disease (representing the "residual" effects of better health-care strategies overall), are becoming increasingly apparent. The most obvious example of this phenomenon is the increasing burden of chronic heart failure.

1

It is within this context that this chapter describes the epidemiology and probable burden of heart failure during the first few decades of the twenty-first century.

The increasing burden of heart failure

Chronic heart failure is now recognised as a major and escalating public health problem in industrialised countries with ageing populations. However, determining its current burden on individual countries remains problematic. This uncertainty is the product of two related problems. First, heart failure represents a complex pathological process that is the terminal manifestation of a number of diverse cardiac disease states (from coronary heart disease through valve disease, endocardial and pericardial problems to idiopathic cardiomyopathy, to list just a few). As such, it is associated with a broad spectrum of clinical presentations and defies simple definition. Second, to date there has been no large-scale, systematic investigation of the epidemiology of chronic heart failure from both a physiological and a clinical perspective within the same population. The majority of epidemiological data relate to the "symptomatic" syndrome of heart failure and there are undoubtedly many asymptomatic patients who might be legitimately labelled with a diagnosis of "heart failure" (for example, those with asymptomatic left ventricular systolic dysfunction). The symptomatic syndrome of chronic heart failure is usually characterised by the following:

- left ventricular dysfunction
- abnormal neurohormonal regulation
- unmet metabolic demand
- breathlessness and intolerance to exercise
- fluid retention
- premature death.

Data relating to the aetiology, epidemiology, and prognostic implications of chronic heart failure are principally available from five types of studies:

- cross-sectional and longitudinal follow-up surveys of well-defined populations: these have almost exclusively focused on individuals with clinical signs and symptoms indicative of chronic congestive heart failure
- cross-sectional surveys of individuals who have been medically treated for signs and symptoms of heart failure within a well-defined region
- echocardiographic surveys of individuals within a well-defined population to determine the prevalence of left ventricular systolic dysfunction
- nationwide studies of annual trends in hospitalisation related to heart failure identified on the basis of diagnostic coding at discharge
- comprehensive clinical trial and trial registry data sets: these include a

large proportion of individuals who were identified on the basis of having both impaired left ventricular systolic dysfunction and signs and symptoms of heart failure.

Within the context of the specific limitations of the type of data available, and the inherent bias towards describing chronic congestive heart failure secondary to left ventricular systolic dysfunction, the following sections describe the modern-day burden of chronic heart failure.

The epidemiology of heart failure

Prevalence

Table 1.1 is a summary of the reported prevalence of heart failure according to whether this was estimated from a survey of individuals requiring medical treatment from a general practitioner, or from population screening. Despite the wide variation in the reported overall prevalence of heart failure (largely reflecting different research methodologies and study cohorts), these data demonstrate that the prevalence of heart failure increases markedly with age and that it has become more common in the last few decades of the twentieth century.

Table 1.1 Reported prevalence of heart failure.

Study	Location	Prevalence rate, (whole population) (/1000)	Prevalence rate in older age-groups (/1000)
Surveys of treated patients			
Logan et al. (1958)[3]	National data (RCGP), UK	3	–
Gibson et al. (1966)[4]	Rural cohort, USA	9–10	65 (> 65 yr)
RCGP (1988)[5]	National data, UK	11	–
Parameshwar et al. (1992)[6]	London, UK	4	28 (> 65 yr)
Rodeheffer (1993)[7]	Rochester, USA	3 (< 75 yr)	–
Mair et al. (1996)[8]	Liverpool, UK	15	80 (> 65 yr)
RCGP (1995)[9]	National data, UK	9	74 (65–74 yr)
Clarke et al. (1995)[10]	Nottinghamshire, UK	8–16	40–60 (> 70 yr)
Population screening			
Droller and Pemberton (1953)[11]	Sheffield, UK	–	30–50 (> 62 yr)
Garrison et al. (1966)[12]	Georgia, USA	21 (45–74 yr)	35 (65–74 yr)
McKee et al. (1971)[13]	Framingham, USA	3 (< 63 yrs)	23 (60–79 yr)
Landahl et al. (1984)[14]	Sweden (males only)	3 (< 75 yr)	80–170 (> 67 yr)
Eriksson et al. (1989)[15]	Gothenburg, Sweden	–	130 (> 67 yr)
Schocken et al.[16]	NHANES data, USA	20	80/1000 (> 65 yr)
RCGP (1995)[9]	National data, UK	9 (25–74 yr)	74 (65–74 yr)

Studies of patients visiting a general practitioner

In the UK there have been a number of large studies examining the prevalence of patients being treated for heart failure by a general practitioner. For example, in 1992, Parameshwar and colleagues[6] examined the clinical records of diuretic-treated patients in three general practices in north-west London. From a total of 30 204 patients, a clinical diagnosis of heart failure was made in 117 cases (46 men and 71 women), giving an overall prevalence rate of 3.9 cases per 1000. Prevalence increased markedly with age – in those aged under 65 years the prevalence rate was 0.6 cases per 1000 compared with 28 cases per 1000 in those aged over 65 years. However, objective investigation of left ventricular function had been undertaken in less than one-third of these patients. In 1995, Clarke and colleagues[10] reported an even larger survey of chronic heart failure based on similar methods and including analysis of loop diuretic prescriptions for all residents of Nottinghamshire. They estimated that between 13 017 and 26 214 patients had been prescribed frusemide. Case-note review of a random sample of patients receiving such treatment found that 56% were being treated for heart failure. On this basis an overall prevalence rate was calculated of 8–16 per 1000. Once again, prevalence increased with advancing age, with the rate increasing to 40–60 cases per 1000 among those aged over 70 years.

Population studies based on clinical criteria

The National Health and Nutrition Examination Survey (NHANES-I)[16] reported the prevalence of heart failure within the US population. Based on self-reporting, and using a clinical scoring system, this study screened 14 407 men and women aged 25–47 years between 1971 and 1975, with detailed evaluation of only 6 913 subjects and reported a prevalence rate of 20 cases per 1000. The Helsinki Ageing Study described clinical and echocardiographic findings in 501 subjects (367 female) aged 75–86 years.[17] Prevalence of heart failure, based on clinical criteria, was 8.2% overall (41 of 501) and 6.8%, 10%, and 8.1% in those aged 75, 80 and 85 years respectively. As might be expected in an elderly population with a clinical diagnosis of heart failure, there was a high prevalence of moderate or severe mitral or aortic valvular disease (51%), ischaemic heart disease (54%), and hypertension (54%). However, of the 41 subjects with "heart failure", only 11 had significant left ventricular systolic dysfunction (diagnosed by fractional shortening or left ventricular dilatation) and in 20 subjects no echocardiographic abnormality was identified. Despite this, the 4-year relative risks of all-cause and cardiovascular mortality associated with chronic heart failure in this population were 2.1 and 4.2, respectively.

4

Major limitation of estimating heart failure prevalence using clinical criteria alone

In only a few of the studies described above was objective evidence of cardiac dysfunction (for example, chest radiography) obtained. Consequently, it is unclear whether all patients really had heart failure and, if they did, what the cause of heart failure was. Moreover, patients with heart failure and impaired left ventricular ejection fraction often do not have radiographic cardiomegaly.

Prevalence of left ventricular systolic dysfunction

Three estimates of the population prevalence of left ventricular systolic dysfunction as determined by echocardiography have emanated from Scotland,[18] The Netherlands,[19] and England.[20] The Scottish study targeted a representative cohort of 2000 persons aged 25–74 years. Of those selected, 1640 (82%) had a detailed assessment of their cardiovascular status and underwent echocardiography. Left ventricular systolic dysfunction was defined as a left ventricular ejection fraction of 30% or less. The overall prevalence of left ventricular systolic dysfunction using this criterion was 2.9%. Concurrent symptoms of heart failure were found in 1.5% of the cohort, whilst the remaining 1.4% were asymptomatic. Prevalence was greater in men and increased with age (in men aged 65–74 years it was 6.4% and in age-matched women it was 4.9%).[21] The Rotterdam study in The Netherlands, though examining individuals aged 55–74 years, reported similar findings. Overall the prevalence of left ventricular systolic dysfunction, defined in this case as fractional shortening of 25% or less, was 5.5% in men and 2.2% in women.[19] More recently, Morgan and colleagues[20] studied 817 individuals aged 70–84 years selected from two general practices in Southampton, England. Left ventricular function was assessed qualitatively as normal, mild, moderate, or severe dysfunction. The overall prevalence of all grades of dysfunction was 7.5% (95% CI, 5.8 to 9.5%). Prevalence of left ventricular dysfunction doubled between the age ranges of 70–74 years and over 80 years.

Incidence

Much less is known about the incidence of heart failure compared with its prevalence. The most detailed incidence data emanates from The Framingham Heart Study.[21] This study is based on the periodic screening of a small, geographically selected semiurban population in the USA. As with the population-based prevalence studies, heart failure was defined according to a clinical scoring system. The only "cardiac" investigation was a chest radiograph. After 34 years of follow-up, the incidence rate was approximately 2 cases per 1000 in those aged 45–54 years, increasing to 40 cases per 1000 in men aged 85–94 years.[13, 22] Using similar criteria, Eriksson and colleagues[15] reported incidence rates of "manifest" heart failure of 1.5, 4.3, and 10.2 cases per 1000, in men aged 50–54, 55–60 and 61–67 years respectively. More recently, Rodeheffer and colleagues[7] also reported the incidence of heart failure in a US population residing in Rochester during 1981 in persons aged 0–74 years. The annual incidence was 1.1 cases per 1000. Once again the incidence was higher in men than in women (1.57 versus 0.71 cases per 1000). It also increased with age – new cases increasing from 0.76 male cases per 1000 in those aged 45–49 years to 1.6 male cases per 1000 in those aged 65–69 years.

Cowie and colleagues reported an incidence study from a district of London with a population of approximately 150 000. In a 15-month period, 122 patients were referred to a special heart failure clinic, representing an annual referral rate of 6.5 cases per 1000 population. Using a broad definition of heart failure, only 29% of these patients were clearly diagnosed as having heart failure (annual incidence 1.85 per 1000 population).[23] Table 1.2 summarises the data from the major incidence studies.

Table 1.2 Reported incidence of heart failure.

Study	Location	Incidence rate, (whole population) (/1000)	Incidence rate in older age-groups (/1000)
Eriksson *et al.* (1989)[15]	Sweden (men born in 1913)	–	10 (61–67yr)
Remes *et al.* (1992)[24]	Eastern Finland	1–4 (45–74 yr)	8 (> 65 yr)
Ho *et al.* (1993)[22]	Framingham, USA	2	–
Rodeheffer *et al.* (1993)[7]	Rochester, USA	1 (< 75 yr)	16 (> 65 yr)
Cowie *et al.* (1999)[23]	London, UK	1	12 (> 85 yr)

Hospitalisation rates

Some of the most reliable epidemiological data on heart failure come from reports of hospital admissions on a country-by-country basis: although these need to be interpreted with some caution owing to their retrospective nature, variations in coding practices, and changing admission thresholds over time. Figure 1.1 compares reported hospitalisation rates from Scotland,[25] Spain,[26] the USA,[27, 28] Sweden,[29] New Zealand,[30] and The Netherlands.[31] The number of heart failure admissions in each of these countries was reported to be increasing. For example, studies undertaken in the UK suggest that 0.2% of the population in the early 1990s were hospitalised for heart failure per annum, and that such admissions accounted for more than 5% of adult general medicine and geriatric hospital admissions – outnumbering those associated with acute myocardial infarction.[32] In the USA heart failure is the most common cause of hospitalisation in people over the age of 65 years.[28] The duration of hospital stay is frequently prolonged and in many cases is rapidly followed by readmission. For example, in the UK the mean length of stay for a heart failure-related hospitalisation in 1990 was 11.4 days on acute medical wards and 28.5 days on acute geriatric wards.[25] Within the UK about one-third of patients are readmitted within 12 months of discharge, whilst the same proportion are reported to be readmitted within 6 months in the USA.[27, 28] Such readmission rates are usually higher than the other major causes of hospitalisation, including stroke, hip fracture, and respiratory disease.[32] On a sex-specific basis, men tend to be younger than women when admitted for the first time with heart failure, but because of greater female longevity, the number of male and female admissions are roughly equal. Moreover, the average age of a first admission for heart failure appears to be increasing.[33]

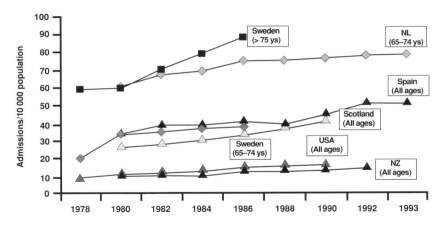

Figure 1.1 Comparison of heart failure admissions rates per annum (recorded hospital admissions per 10000 population at risk) in six industrialised countries 1978–1993.

Cost of heart failure

In any health-care system, hospitalisations represent a disproportionate component of total health-care expenditure. The overall management of heart failure consumes a significant amount (1–2%) of health-care expenditure in developed countries (Figure 1.2).[29, 30, 32, 34–36] Moreover, the increasing˜ rates of hospitalisation make it likely that these reported estimates fall short of the current economic burden.

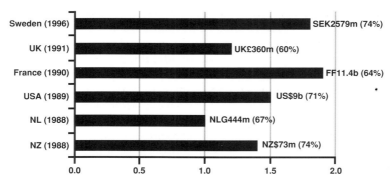

Figure 1.2 The cost of chronic heart failure compared with total health-care expenditure in six industrialised countries. Percentages shown in parentheses represent the proportion of expenditure relating to hospital-based costs (FF, French francs; NLG, Netherlands guilders; SEK, Swedish kronor; b, billion; m, million).

Aetiology of heart failure

Coronary heart disease, either alone or in combination with hypertension, seems to be the most common cause of heart failure. It is, however, difficult to be certain what is the primary reason for heart failure in a patient with multiple potential causes. Furthermore, even the absence of overt hypertension in a patient presenting with heart failure does not rule out an important aetiological role in the past, with normalisation of blood pressure as the patient develops pump failure. Even in those with suspected coronary heart disease the diagnosis is not always correct.

Some of the more common precursors of chronic heart failure include:

- coronary heart disease (consequent upon acute myocardial infarction)
- chronic hypertension
- cardiomyopathy (dilated, hypertrophic, alcoholic and idiopathic)
- valvular dysfunction (diseases of the aortic or mitral valve)
- cardiac arrhythmias/conduction disturbance (heart block and atrial fibrillation)
- pericardial disease (constrictive pericarditis)
- infection (rheumatic fever, Chagas disease, viral myocarditis and HIV).

In the initial cohort of the Framingham Heart Study monitored until 1965, hypertension appeared to be the most common cause of heart failure, being identified as the primary cause in 30% of men and 20% of women and a cofactor in a further 33% and 25% cases respectively.[37] Furthermore, electrocardiographic evidence of left ventricular hypertrophy in the presence of hypertension carried an approximately 15-fold increased risk for the development of heart failure. In the subsequent years of follow-up, however, coronary heart disease became increasingly prevalent prior to the development of heart failure and, as the identified cause of new cases of heart failure, increased from 22% in the 1950s to almost 70% in the 1970s. During this period the relative contribution of hypertension and valvular heart disease declined dramatically: per decade, there was a decline in the prevalence of hypertension during this period of approximately 5% in men and 30% in women.[38] The declining contribution of hypertension most probably reflects the introduction of antihypertensive therapy; the parallel decline in the prevalence of left ventricular hypertrophy supports this supposition. It is also probable that during this same period, progressively greater accuracy in identifying the presence of coronary heart disease contributed to its increasing importance in this regard.

Any interpretation of the Framingham data has to consider the fact that heart failure was identified on clinical criteria alone and undoubtedly included individuals without associated left ventricular systolic dysfunction. Conversely, the large-scale clinical trials mostly recruited patients who had a reduced left ventricular ejection fraction, and applied an extensive list of exclusion criteria. Table 1.3 is a summary of the most common attributed causes and associations of heart failure in a number of clinical trials and registers.[39–45]

Table 1.3 Aetiology of heart failure in clinical trials and registers.[39–46]

	Clinical trials					Registers	
	SOLVD	DIG Study	MERIT-HF	ATLAS	RALES	SOLVD	SPICE
	1991	1997	1999	1999	1999	1992	1999
Size of cohort	2569	6800	3991	3192	1663	6273	9580
Mean age	61	64	64	64	65	62	66
Male (%)	80	78	78	79	73	74	74
Aetiology of heart failure							
Ischaemic (%)	71	70	66	64	54	69	63
Non-ischaemic (%)		29	34	35	46	31	–
Hypertensive (%)	–	(9)	–	(20)	–	7	4
Idiopathic cardiomyopathy (%)	18	(15)	–	(28)	–	13	17
Valvular (%)	–	–	–	(6)	–	–	5
Other (%)	–	6	–	–	–	11	–
Unknown (%)	–	–	–	–	–	–	6
Comorbidity							
Hypertension (%)	42	–	44	46	–	43	27
Diabetes (%)	26	–	25	29	–	23	–
Atrial fibrillation (%)	10	–	17	–	–	14	–
Current angina (%)	37	–	–	27	–	–	
Respiratory disease (%)	26	–	–	–	–	15	–

In a study of left ventricular function in western Scotland, 95% versus 71% of symptomatic and asymptomatic individuals with definite left ventricular systolic dysfunction had evidence of coronary heart disease (p = 0.04). Individuals with symptomatic heart failure were also more likely to have a past myocardial infarction (50% versus 14%; p = 0.01) and concurrent angina (62% v 43%; p = 0.02). Hypertension (80%) and valvular heart disease (25%) were also more prevalent in individuals with both clinical and echocardiographically determined heart failure compared with the remainder of the cohort – including those with asymptomatic left ventricular dysfunction (67% and 0% respectively).[18]

Therefore, the aetiological importance of many of the associated causes of heart failure will depend both on the age cohorts examined, and the type of criteria used to determine the presence of heart failure.

Prognostic implications of chronic heart failure

Chronic heart failure, irrespective of whether it has been detected in patients being actively treated (for example, during hospitalisation) or in otherwise asymptomatic individuals, is a lethal condition. Mortality rates may be comparable to that of cancer. For example, in the original and subsequent Framingham cohorts, the probability of someone dying within 5 years of being diagnosed with heart failure was 62% and 75% in men and 38% and 42% in women respectively. In comparison, 5-year survival for all cancers among men and women in the USA during the same period was approximately 50%.[46] The general applicability of these data is limited by the few events recorded overall, the relative homogeneity of the Framingham population, and the exclusion of older individuals.

The Rochester epidemiology project has described the prognosis in 107 patients presenting to associated hospitals with new-onset heart failure in 1981, and 141 patients presenting in 1991.[47] The median duration of follow-up in these cohorts was 1061 and 1233 days respectively. The mean age of the 1981 patients was 75 years rising to 77 years in 1991. The 1-year and 5-year mortality rates were, respectively, 28% and 66% in the 1981 cohort, and 23% and 67% in the 1991 cohort. In other words, although the same diagnostic criteria used in the Framingham study were used in the Rochester project, the prognosis was somewhat better in the latter.

The only other large, representative, epidemiological study reporting long-term outcome in patients with heart failure is the NHANES-I survey.[16] The initial programme evaluated 14 407 adults aged 25–74 years in the USA between 1971 and 1975. Follow-up studies were carried out in 1982–4 and again in 1986 (for those aged 55 years or over and alive during the 1982–4 review). The estimated 10-year mortality in subjects aged 25–74 years with self-reported heart failure was 42.8% (49.8% in men and 36% in women). Mortality in those aged 65–74 years was 65.4% (71.8%

in men and 59.5% in women). These mortality rates are considerably lower than those observed in Framingham. However, the patients in NHANES-I were non-institutionalised; their heart failure was self-reported and follow-up was incomplete. This investigation was also more recent than the Framingham study, and the prognosis for heart failure may have improved; although neither study reported an improved prognostic outlook for heart failure over time.

Despite careful selection (predominantly otherwise healthy younger men), 'gold standard' pharmacotherapy, and careful management, the mortality rates among participants in clinical trials have also been reportedly high. For example, during 10-year follow-up of the original CONSENSUS-1 cohort ($n = 253$) only 5 patients were found to be alive.[48] During a mean follow-up of 41 months in the SOLVD study treatment arm a total of 962 patients died (39.7% in the placebo group and 35.2% in the enalapril treatment group).[44] The true contribution of heart failure to overall mortality or coronary heart disease-related mortality is almost certainly underestimated. Although heart failure is highly prevalent among the elderly, is the end-product of a number of cardiovascular disease states, and has been shown to be associated with extremely poor survival rates, official statistics continue to attribute only a small proportion of deaths to this condition. A study of Scottish death data during the period 1979–92, showed that while heart failure was recorded as the underlying cause of death in only 1.5% of cases, it was found to be a contributory cause in an additional 14.3% of deaths.[49] Importantly, this study demonstrated that one-third of coronary heart disease-related deaths may have been due to heart failure.

Quality of life

Two large studies from the USA have shown that heart failure impairs self-reported quality of life more than any other common chronic medical disorder.[50, 51] Quality of life deteriorates with increasing heart failure severity, and this is associated with increased numbers of physician visits, drug consumption, and hospitalisation. The prevalence of major depression in a hospitalised cohort of chronically patients aged over 60 years was found to be significantly greater in those with chronic heart failure (36.5% versus 25.5% for the remaining cohort). Such depression was both prolonged and largely untreated in the chronic heart failure cohort.[52]

Health-related quality of life is being increasingly recognised as an important end-point in trials of both pharmacological and non-pharmacological treatment strategies. Rather than solely measuring duration of survival, studies are being designed with a quality of life component in order to determine whether greater longevity equates to

11

poor quality of life before an inevitable death. As the focus on the individual patient becomes more important, quality of life measures are even being incorporated into primary end-points, rather than being measured as a secondary end-point: particularly when examining strategies where prolonging survival is not the principal concern. It should be noted, however, that many hospitalised patients with severe heart failure would still prefer to be resuscitated if required.[53]

The future of heart failure

As noted above, despite an overall decline in age-adjusted mortality from coronary heart disease in developed countries overall, the number of these patients is increasing.[1] This reflects a higher proportion of older individuals, in whom incidence of coronary heart disease and hypertension is highest,[54] and improved overall survival rates overall. In particular, survival after acute myocardial infarction increased markedly in the UK during the 1990s, at least in part because of better medical treatment.[33] As coronary heart disease is the most powerful risk factor for heart failure, it is likely that the aforementioned trends will lead to an increase in its prevalence in the future. It will probably become, therefore, a more common manifestation of chronic coronary heart disease, as well as contributing to an increasing number of deaths. Two formal projections of the future burden of heart failure have been undertaken in respect to Australia[1] and The Netherlands.[54] Figure 1.3 shows the projected number of cases of heart failure within the relatively small population of Australia (approximately 18 million people). The projected increases are certainly dramatic. Likewise, an analysis of demographic trends in The Netherlands has predicted that the prevalence of heart failure, due to coronary heart disease, will rise by 70% during the period 1985 to 2010.[1]

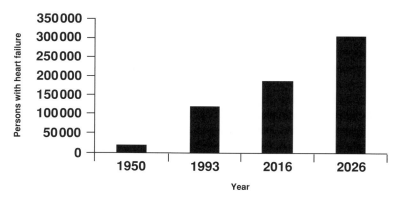

Figure 1.3 Increasing burden of heart failure among those aged 65 years and over in Australia.

Conclusion

Heart failure represents a growing health problem. Currently available pharmacological treatment strategies do not completely ameliorate the high morbidity and mortality rates associated with chronic heart failure – especially in older individuals. There is a clear need to develop and implement cost-effective programmes that prevent the development of heart failure (for example, primary prevention in coronary heart disease). There is also a need for programmes that provide for the early detection and treatment of individuals who develop heart failure despite prevention strategies (for example, screening with echocardiography).

Unfortunately, the most urgent need relates to the increasing number of older individuals with chronic heart failure who are being hospitalised. Such individuals have limited survival prospects and are likely to have an extremely poor quality of life and require recurrent hospitalisation before they die. It is within this context that specialist nurse intervention programmes have the potential to alleviate the overall burden of chronic heart failure by limiting costly hospital admissions, in addition to improving quality of life on an individual basis by providing more tailored and attentive health care.

References

1 Kelly DT. Our future society: a global challenge. *Circulation* 1997; **95**: 2459–64.
2 Caselli G, Lopez AD. *Health and mortality among elderly populations.* New York: Clarendon Press, 1996.
3 Logan WPD, Cushion AA. *Morbidity statistics from general practice*, vol. 1. Studies on Medical and Population Subjects No. 14. London: HSMO, 1958.
4 Gibson TC, White KL, Klainer LM. The prevalence of congestive heart failure in two rural communities. *J Chron Dis* 1966; **19**: 141–52.
5 Royal College of General Practitioners, Office of Population Censuses and Surveys, and Department of Health and Social Security. *Morbidity statistics from general practice: third national study, 1981–82.* London: HMSO, 1988.
6 Parameshwar J, Shackell MM, Richardson A, Poole-Wilson PA, Sutton GC. Prevalence of heart failure in three general practices in north west London. Br J Gen Pract 1992; **42**: 287–9.
7 Rodeheffer RJ, Jacobsen SJ, Gersh BJ, *et al.* The incidence and prevalence of congestive heart failure in Rochester, Minnesota. *Mayo Clin Proc* 1993; **68**: 1143–50.
8 Mair FS, Crowley TS, Bundred PE. Prevalence, aetiology and management of heart failure in general practice. *Br J Gen Prac* 1996; **46**: 77–9.
9 Royal College of General Practitioners, Office of Population Censuses and Surveys, and Department of Health and Social Security. *Morbidity statistics from general practice: fourth national study, 1991–92.* London: HMSO, 1995.
10 Clarke KW, Gray D, Hampton JR. How common is heart failure? Evidence from PACT (Prescribing Analysis and Cost) data in Nottingham. *J Publ Health Med* 1995; **17**: 459–64.
11 Droller H, Pemberton J. Cardiovascular disease in a random sample of elderly people. *Br Heart J* 1953; **15**: 199–204.
12 Garrison GE, McDonough JR, Hames CG, Stulb SC. Prevalence of chronic congestive heart failure in the population of Evans County, Georgia. *Am J Epidemiol* 1966; **83**: 338–44.
13 McKee PA, Castelli WP, McNamara PM, Kannel WB. The natural history of congestive

heart failure: the Framingham study. *N Engl J Med* 1971; **285**: 1441–46.

14　Landahl S, Svanborg A, Astrand K. Heart volume and the prevalence of certain common cardiovascular disorders at 70 and 75 years of age. *Eur Heart J* 1984; **5**: 326–31.

15　Eriksson H, Svardsudd K, Larsson B *et al.* Risk factors for heart failure in the general population: the study of men born in 1913. *Eur Heart J* 1989; **10**: 647–56.

16　Schocken DD, Arrieta MI, Leaverton PE, Ross EA. Prevalence and mortality rate of congestive heart failure in the United States. *J Am Coll Cardiol* 1992; **20**: 301–6.

17　Kupari M, Lindroos M, Iivanainen AM, Heikkila J, Tilvis R. Congestive heart failure in old age: prevalence, mechanisms and 4-year prognosis in the Helsinki ageing study. *J Int Med* 1997; **241**: 387–94.

18　McDonagh TA, Morrison CE, Lawrence A *et al.* Symptomatic and asymptomatic left-ventricular systolic dysfunction in an urban population. 1997; **350**: 829–33.

19　Mosterd A, de Bruijne MC, Hoes AW *et al.* Usefulness of echocardiography in detecting left ventricular dysfunction in population based studies (The Rotterdam Study). *Am J Cardiol* 1997; **79**: 103–4.

20　Morgan S, Smith H, Simpson I *et al.* Prevalence and clinical characteristics of left ventricular dysfunction among elderly patients in general practice setting: cross sectional survey. *Br Med J* 1999; **318**: 368–72

21　Margolis JR, Gillum RF, Feinleb M, Brasch RC, Fabsitz RR. Community surveillance for coronary heart disease: the Framingham Cardiovascular Disease Study. Methods and preliminary results. *Am J Epidemiol* 1974; **100**: 425–36.

22　Ho KK, Pinsky JL, Kannel WB, Levy D. The epidemiology of heart failure: the Framingham Study. *J Am Coll Cardiol* 1993; **22**: 6A–13A.

23　Cowie MR, Wood DA, Coats AJ *et al.* Incidence and aetiology of heart failure: a population-based study. *Eur Heart J* 1999; **20**: 421–8.

24　Remes J, Reunanen A, Aromaa A, Pyorala A. Incidence of heart failure in eastern Finland: a population-based surveillance study. *Eur Heart J* 1992; **13**: 588–93.

25　McMurray J, McDonagh T, Morrison CE, Dargie HJ. Trends in hospitalization for heart failure in Scotland 1980–1990. *Eur Heart J* 1993; **14**: 1158–62.

26　Rodriguez-Artalejo F, Guallar-Castillon P, Banegas Banegas JR, del Rey Calero J. Trends in hospitalization and mortality for heart failure in Spain, 1980-1993. *Eur Heart J* 1997; **18**: 1771–9.

27　Ghali JK, Cooper R, Ford E. Trends in hospitalisation rates for heart failure in the United States 1973-1986: evidence for screening population prevalence. *Arch Intern Med* 1992; **150**: 769–73.

28　Haldeman GA, Croft JB, Giles WH, Rashidee A. Hospitalization of patients with heart failure: national hospital discharge survey 1985–1995. *Am Heart J* 1999; **137**: 352–60.

29　Eriksson H, Wilhelmsen L, Caidahl K, Svardsudd K. Epidemiology and prognosis of heart failure. *Z Kardiol* 1991; **80**: 1–6.

30　Doughty R, Yee T, Sharpe N *et al.* Hospital admissions and deaths due to congestive heart failure in New Zealand, 1988-91. *NZ Med J* 1995; **108**: 473–5.

31　Reitsma JB, Mosterd A, de Craen AJM *et al.* Increase in hospital admission rates for heart failure in the Netherlands, 1980–1993. *Heart* 1996; **76**: 388–92.

32　Murray J, Hart W, Rhodes G. An evaluation of the cost of heart failure to the National Health Service in the UK. *Br J Med Econ* 1993; **6**: 91–8.

33　K MacIntyre, Capewell S, Livingston J *et al.* Mortality trends in 86,000 patients admitted with heart failure, 1981–1995 [Abstract]. *Eur Heart J* 1999; **20**: S257.

34　Launois R, Launois B, Reboul-Marty J *et al.* Le coût de la sévérité de la maladie: le cas de l'insuffisance-cardiaque. *J Econ Med* 1990; **8**: 395–412.

35　Van Hout BA, Wielink G, Bonsel GJ *et al.* Effects of ACE inhibitors on heart failure in The Netherlands: a pharmacoeconomic model. *PharmacoEconomics* 1993; **3**: 387–97.

36　Konstam M, Dracup K, Baker D *et al. Heart failure: evaluation and care of patients with left ventricular systolic dysfunction.* Clinical Practice Guideline No. 11. AHCPR Publication No 94-0612 Rockville, MD: Agency for Health Care Policy and Research, Public Health Service, US Department of Health and Human Services, June 1994.

37　Levy D, Larson MG, Vasan RS, Kannel WB, Ho KL. The progression from hypertension to congestive heart failure. *JAMA* 1996; **275**: 1557–62.

38　Kannel WB, Ho KK, Thom T. Changing epidemiological features of cardiac failure. *Eur Heart J* 1994; **72**: S3–9.

39 The SOLVD Investigators. Effect of enalapril on survival in patients with reduced left ventricular ejection fractions and congestive heart failure. *N Engl J Med* 1991; **325**: 293–302.

40 Pitt B, Zannad F, Remme WJ *et al.* The effect of spironolactone on morbidity and mortality in patients with severe heart failure. Randomized Aldactone Evaluation Study Investigators. *N Engl J Med* 1999; **341**: 709–17.

41 The Digitalis Investigation Group. The effect of digoxin on mortality and morbidity in patients with heart failure. *N Engl J Med* 1997; **336**: 525–33.

42 MERIT Investigators. Effect of metoprolol CR/XL in chronic heart failure: Metoprolol CR/XL Randomised Intervention Trial in Congestive Heart Failure (Merit-HF). *Lancet* 1999; **353**: 2001–7.

43 Packer M, Poole-Wilson PA, Armstrong PW *et al.* Comparative effects of low and high doses of the angiotensin converting enzyme inhibitor, lisinopril, on morbidity and mortality in chronic heart failure. *Circulation* 1999; **100**: 2312-18.

44 SOLVD Investigators. Natural history and patterns of current practice in heart failure. *J Am Coll Cardiol* 1993; **4A**: 14A–19A.

45 Bart BA, Ertl G, Held P *et al.* Contemporary management of patients with left ventricular systolic dysfunction. Results from the study of patients intolerant of converting enzyme inhibitors (SPICE) registry. *Eur Heart J* 1999; **20**: 1182–90.

46 Ho KKL, Anderson KM, Karmel WB *et al.* Survival after the onset of congestive heart failure in the Framingham Heart Study subjects. *Circulation* 1993; **88**: 107–15.

47 Senni M, Tribouilloy CM, Rodeheffer RJ *et al.* Congestive heart failure in the community – trends in incidence and survival in a 10-year period. *Arch Intern Med* 1999; **159**: 29–34.

48 Swedberg K, Kjekshus J, Snapinn S. Long-term survival in severe heart failure in patients treated with enalapril. Ten year follow-up of CONSENSUS 1. *Eur Heart J* 1999; **2**: 136–9.

49 Murdoch DR, Love MP, Robb SD. Importance of heart failure as a cause of death: contribution to overall mortality and coronary heart disease mortality in Scotland 1979–1992. *Eur Heart J* 1998; **19**: 1829–35.

50 Stewart AL, Greenfield S, Hays RD *et al.* Functional status and well-being of patients with chronic conditions – results from the medical outcomes study. *JAMA* 1989; **262**: 907–13.

51 Fryback DG, Dasbach EJ, Klein R *et al.* The Beaver Dam Health Outcomes Study – initial catalog of health-state quality factors. *Med Dec Making* 1993; **13**: 89–102.

52 Koenig HG. Depression in hospitalized older patients with congestive heart failure. *Gen Hosp Psych* 1998; **20**: 29–43.

53 Krumholz HM, Phillips RS, Hamel MB *et al.* Resuscitation preferences among patients with severe congestive heart failure: results from the SUPPORT project. *Circulation* 1998; **98**: 648–55.

54 Bonneux L, Barendregt JJ, Meeter K *et al.* Estimating clinical morbidity due to ischaemic heart disease and congestive heart failure: the future rise of heart failure. *Am J Publ Health* 1994; **84**: 20-8.

2: Determinants of health-care utilisation by patients with chronic heart failure

TINY JAARSMA, KATHLEEN DRACUP

Heart failure is the leading cause of hospital admission for patients over the age of 65 years in most industrialised countries.[1-6] In the USA, the period 1973–86 saw an increase of more than 50% in hospitalisations, with comparable trends in Europe. Heart failure has become a significant public health problem, with a rapid rise in incidence and prevalence that is predicted to continue well into the future.[7, 8]

Longer survival of patients with heart disease and more complete and accurate reporting have been cited as leading reasons for the rise in hospitalisation rates for heart failure patients.[3] Reported hospitalisation rates indicate that patients with heart failure have the highest readmission rates of all patients.[9] Recurrent heart failure is the most common cause for readmission and is often unavoidable.[9, 10] However, other factors contributing to readmission include new medical problems (arrhythmias, hypertension, stroke), non-compliance with the treatment regimen, adverse reactions to medications, use of detrimental drug therapy (for example, class Ic antiarrhythmic agents, non-steroidal anti-inflammatory agents, first-generation calcium antagonists), and problems with caregivers or extended care facilities.[11-13] Several investigators have concluded that readmissions would have been avoided in 40–59% of patients if there had been better assessments, if rehabilitation had been more adequate, if discharge had been more carefully planned, if potential non-compliance problems with medications and diet had been identified, and if patients had been instructed to seek medical attention when symptoms first occurred.[10, 14-16] Yet, despite a well structured multidisciplinary approach and careful discharge planning, it is estimated that at least 8% of all patients discharged with a diagnosis of heart failure still will be readmitted within 3 months.[17]

In this chapter the determinants for readmission to the emergency room and hospital for patients with heart failure are discussed.

Patient-related factors

Sociodemographic factors

Although there is no single sociodemographic profile that predicts high resource utilisation in heart failure patients, different factors are independently related to hospital readmission rates.[10, 15, 18–21] These factors can be used to design and tailor interventions to specific patient groups, such as targeting interventions to frail, elderly patients with heart failure or to female patients. However, sociodemographic and clinical factors are often interrelated. For example, older people tend to live alone, or with an elderly spouse who often also has a health problem, thus reducing available social resources. Sociodemographic variables related to increased health-care resource use include age, sex, ethnicity, socioeconomic status, and social support.

Age

Although age is not an independent predictor of readmission in most studies, heart failure patients are elderly and more vulnerable to poorer outcomes.[11, 22, 23] As a consequence they are readmitted to the hospital or emergency department more often than younger patients.[15, 18, 24] Thus, it is important to consider factors that are related to readmission in the elderly. Compared with younger patients, older patients who visit the emergency room or who are hospitalised present more often with life-threatening or urgent medical conditions, and have a complaint related to self-care, falls, or social issues. Older patients require a greater number of tests and other resources, have longer hospital stays, and have several comorbidities.[25] Older patients often have decreased renal function and a reduced ability to excrete drugs in the active form; they are thus are more vulnerable to adverse drug reactions than younger patients, which often leads to rehospitalisation.

Sex

Relatively little is known about the effect of the patients sex on clinical presentation and outcome, since few women are enrolled in heart failure studies. Compared with men with heart failure, women with the disease are often older, have a higher prevalence of hypertension and diabetes, and have a lower prevalence of ischaemic heart disease. They also have better survival rates.[1, 26–28] The effect of gender on readmission rates is unclear. In two studies of elderly patients with heart failure, men were much more likely to be readmitted than women.[22, 29] However, in a study of a cohort of heart failure patients younger than 60 years, African-American women were at increased risk for hospitalisation for heart failure.[30] Women patients also tend to have a longer duration of hospital stay, often leading to increased costs.[28]

Race and ethnicity

Another factor to consider in resource utilisation is the race and cultural background of patients. In a few American studies, the length of stay of African-American patients with heart failure was longer, hospital charges were higher, and mortality and readmission rates were higher compared with white patients.[28, 30] Perhaps differences in the severity and pathophysiology of heart failure can partially account for these variations. Hypertensive heart disease, more common in African-Americans, may result in a more volume-sensitive state, making hypertensive patients more prone to sudden, symptomatic pulmonary congestion and interstitial oedema than patients with heart failure from other causes.[28] Finally, differences in access to adequate health care may result in higher readmission rates for some races.[31, 32]

Socioeconomic status and health insurance

In general, older populations with low income have a high readmission rate.[33] Patients who are poorly insured are more likely to be admitted for heart failure. The relationship between type of insurance and resource utilisation is not clear. Depending on the health-care system, patients with lower socioeconomic status and elderly people commonly have different health insurance coverage from patients with higher socioeconomic status and younger individuals who are still in the workforce. These differences may result in different readmission rates and health-care cost patterns. However, some authors have found that after adjusting for patient characteristics and hospital type and location, care given within a Health Management Organisation in the USA is associated with shorter lengths of stay and lower hospital charges, the latter partially explained by the former. Medicaid patients in the USA have the longest durations of stay, highest hospital charges, and highest heart failure readmission risk.[34]

Social support

Factors such as widowhood and inadequate social support systems influence the probability of hospital readmission.[35, 36] Both emotional support and practical support have a role in preventing unplanned readmission to the hospital or emergency department. Emotional support can be important not only in motivating patients to comply with their treatment regimen, but also in helping patients cope with this chronic and terminal disease. Emotional support involves support received from partners, family, and friends, as well as that from health-care providers.[37–39] Rich *et al*, found that patients with heart failure living with another person tended to be more compliant with their medication regimens than patients living alone.[40]

Practical support includes help with the activities of daily living, preparation of medication and meals, and transportation to doctor's appointment. Reasons for readmission of the elderly with an inadequate support system include failure to involve home health care, prolonged time to next appointment with the physician, inadequate family involvement, failure of the patient to seek medical attention when symptoms occur, failure to obtain prescribed medications, and inadequate diet.[14, 15, 36]

However, it should be noted that caring for someone with heart failure can be a burden. Relatives sometimes are unable to cope with the life-style adjustments required by the medical condition of the patient. The illness may put family roles and material resources under stress, and spouses may not be physically and emotionally capable of caring for the patient.[36] In one study, one-third of the caregivers, most of whom were women, had a cardiovascular illness themselves. The ability to provide care may be impaired if these caregivers have medical limitations or concerns in addition to those of the spouse.[41, 42]

Clinical and psychosocial factors

Systolic/diastolic dysfunction

Although most of the information on resource utilisation in patients with heart failure has been derived from studies of patients with systolic left ventricular dysfunction, some authors have described rehospitalisation patterns of patients with preserved systolic left ventricular function. Compared with those with significant left ventricular systolic dysfunction, these patients are more likely to have lower hospitalisation costs, a shorter hospital stay and fewer readmissions.[29, 43, 44]

Optimal pharmacological therapy has been defined for heart failure patients with systolic dysfunction, but comparable clinical trials are not available to guide therapy for patients with preserved systolic function. As a consequence, effects of medical treatment on readmission rates are not always applicable to patients with preserved left ventricular function.[45]

Comorbidity and disease severity

Many patients with heart failure also suffer from other illnesses, such as diabetes and chronic obstructive pulmonary disease, which in turn increase the length of hospital stay and the number of readmissions.[21, 46, 47] A comorbid illness often means more medication, resulting in not only a more complex medication regimen for the patient, but also an increased risk of deleterious interactions or side effects. An example of this is the use of non-steroidal anti-inflammatory drugs (NSAIDs), which have an effect on prostaglandin pathways and alter renal flow dynamics. This mechanism promotes fluid retention and worsens renal function in patients with heart failure. The benefits and risk of these agents must be carefully considered in the context of heart failure.[48]

Medical history and severity of illness have also been identified as factors contributing to hospital readmission in the elderly.[20, 36] The average patient with heart failure has three significant comorbidities, each of which can result in increased rates of hospital readmission because of disease progression or problems related to treatment.[18] Not surprisingly, investigators have found that patients with more advanced heart failure are more likely to require readmission than those with moderate disease severity. For example, renal failure is a marker of disease severity in heart failure, and patients with impaired renal function (serum creatinine >170 µmol/l) have higher readmission rates than patients with normal renal function.[49]

Functional status is also a measure of disease severity. Patients with better physical fitness (measured by a 6-minute walk) have lower readmission rates than patients with poor physical fitness, and patients whose functional status improved after an exercise programme had fewer hospital readmissions than patients who were not enrolled in an exercise programme.[50, 51]

Psychosocial status

Patients with heart failure may be depressed for many reasons, including declining physical health, role changes, financial insecurity, and social isolation. Depression in patients with heart failure is often underdiagnosed because the symptoms of depression (such as fatigue, sleep disturbance, and anorexia) are commonly mislabelled as symptoms of heart failure.[52, 53] In several retrospective studies, 17–73% of the patients hospitalised with heart failure were depressed.[52, 54] A study from the USA, identified major depression in 37% of the patients, a rate that was significantly higher than in older, medically ill patients without heart failure (26%).[55] Patients with depression have increased more days and a higher mortality rate than patients who are not depressed.[52]

Non-compliance with treatment

Non-compliance with medication regimens, diet changes, or other recommendations such as seeking medical attention when symptoms occur, is recognised as an important factor for early readmission in heart failure patients.[10, 11, 14–16, 36, 56–63] Overall non-compliance rates range from 42%[16] to 64%,[11] with medication non-compliance varying from 15% to 42%.[57, 61, 64, 65] In a study of elderly patients with heart failure, only 55% of the patients could correctly name which medication had been prescribed, 50% were unable to state the prescribed doses, and 64% could not account for what medication was to be taken, i.e. at what time of day and when in relation to meals the medication was to be taken. In their overall assessment the authors found that

27% were not compliant with their prescribed medicine regimen.[65]

In another study on digoxin use, only 10% of the patients filled enough prescriptions to have received adequate treatment.[57] A large proportion of patients who began digoxin substituted it for other medications or consumed substantially less medication than expected in the first year of therapy.[57]

Non-compliance extends to other aspects of the treatment regimen. In one study almost three-quarters of patients did not weigh themselves daily.[66] A second study on the weighing behaviour of heart failure patients showed that only 40% of them weighed themselves every day and recorded their weights when instructed to do so. Reasons why patients did not weigh themselves included not having a scale, forgetfulness, and not remembering being told.[67] Other factors that contribute to non-compliance include misunderstanding of the instructions given by the general practitioner, senility, adverse drug reactions, polypharmacy, running out of medicine, and the patient's perceived lack of need for the medicine.[14, 56, 68]

Factors related to the health-care system

Factors related to the health-care system responsible for relapses of heart failure are identified in 10–21% of relapses.[11, 61] Inadequate quality of care is a preventable cause for readmission and is often traced to the health-care provider.

Health-care provider

Cardiologists and non-cardiologists differ in the number and type of diagnostic tests they order, their medical treatment, and in their decisions about which type of patient they admit to the hospital.[69] In one prospective cohort study, patients who received direct care from cardiologists had lower predicted rates of mortality, shorter length of stay, and better quality of life than patients who were managed by non-cardiologists. In addition, patients who were treated by cardiologists were more likely to receive recommended diagnostic tests and treatments than patients treated by non-cardiologists, although some of these differences – such as the use of angiotensin-converting enzyme (ACE) inhibitors – could be explained by the variation in the case mix.[69] In another study, patients not treated by a cardiologist had up to a seven-fold increased risk of readmission.[70] The continuing widespread disparity in treatment practices represents an important stimulus to the promulgation of clinical guidelines and increased access to specialists for patients with heart failure.

Inadequate quality of care

If the quality of care is substandard, readmission rates can be expected to rise. In a study reported by Weissman, patients with heart failure who were readmitted had a lower quality of care than those who were not readmitted.[71] Similar findings were reported by Fonarov and colleagues, who reported significant decreases in rehospitalisation rates when patients' medications were optimised and hypervolaemia was carefully monitored and treated.[72] Inadequate quality of care can occur at any stage of treatment, from the initial diagnosis to follow-up care.

Inadequate diagnosis

Although guidelines on diagnosing heart failure are available, there is still debate on the value and necessity of different diagnostic tests in some care settings.[59] In the case of the echocardiogram, many patients who are eligible do not receive this test. Investigators in the UK reported that in one setting only one-third of the patients admitted to hospital with a diagnosis of heart failure had ever had an echocardiogram.[73] Other studies link inadequate diagnostic testing to increased hospital readmission rates.[23, 44] Readmission rates among patients without a recent systolic function assessment were higher compared to patients that had a recent echocardiogram.[44] This finding was confirmed by a study on a large population of patients with heart failure in which multivariate analyses showed that patients undergoing echocardiography, exercise stress testing, or cardiac catheterisation were less likely to be readmitted.[23] However, retrospective studies should be interpreted with caution. The lack of an echocardiogram to establish a diagnosis can be indicative of suboptimal treatment, but it can also reflect a decision to withhold maximal aggressive care at the patient's request.[44]

Inadequate treatment

Clinical guidelines for the treatment of heart failure are well established and updated regularly. However, these guidelines are often not implemented in practice. Evidence from Europe and the USA suggests that a large treatment gap exists between recommended therapies for patients with cardiovascular disease and the care that they actually receive. Clinicians can fail to order medications proved to be effective in the treatment of heart failure, or can order them in doses that are ineffective.[59, 74–76] In one study, 17% of patients with heart failure were prescribed inadequate drug therapy and required readmission.[11] In particular, ACE-inhibitors have been shown to improve mortality and morbidity in patients with heart failure, and their under use has been extensively addressed.[75, 77, 78] Readmission rates are proved to be lower when using proper doses of ACE inhibitors.[79] The CONSENSUS study observed a 28% reduction in hospitalisation with the addition of 20 mg per day of enalapril to patients receiving conventional treatment for chronic heart failure.[59] With the addition of 20 mg of enalapril, a 30% hospital readmission rate was documented.[80] Despite the compelling evidence about ACE inhibitor use, it appears that a significant portion of eligible patients are not receiving these drugs and so are not benefiting from their effects. McMurray summarised the reasons for the low rate of usage of ACE inhibitors as follows:

• failure to recognise that heart failure is an important public health problem worthy of treatment
• failure to appreciate fully the magnitude of the clinical benefit of ACE inhibitors in heart failure
• failure to understand that the clinical benefit of ACE inhibitors fully justifies their cost
• concern that the adverse effects of ACE-inhibitors outweigh their clinical benefits
• belief that the benefits observed in clinical trials does not translate into clinical practice.[75]

Adverse drug reactions

Several studies have linked medication problems to the readmission of patients with heart failure.[14, 15, 36, 81] Medication-related problems include accidental or intentional poisoning, adverse drug reactions, and polypharmacy. Uses of multiple drugs, advanced age, and female sex have been identified as risk factors for developing problems with medications.[82]

Adverse drug effects are a common problem in cardiac patients.[10, 56] For heart failure patients, drug reactions from thiazide diuretics are often the cause of admissions; these agents can cause hypokalaemia with symptoms of nausea, vomiting, and fatigue. Drug interactions and side effects should be carefully monitored and discussed with the patient.

Inadequate patient education

Another vital part of optimal care is patient education. In various clinical guidelines, patient education is recommended as an integral part of care. Topics include general counselling on heart failure, prognosis, activity recommendations, dietary recommendations, medications, and the importance of compliance with the treatment or care plan.[83] The relationship between readmission and patient education is a topic of growing interest. In a study of elderly heart failure patients, lack of patient or family education was related to readmission.[84] In one study conducted by Stewart and colleagues, a teaching programme conducted during a single home visit resulted in a significant reduction in the number of readmissions and days of rehospitalisation.[85] In another study reporting on the effects of a home visit in patients with heart failure, there was no effect on patient compliance.[86] Several heart failure programmes have combined

23

individualised in-hospital patient education with follow-up teaching in the outpatient clinic or home.[62, 72, 86–91] Researchers reported a reduction in the number and length of readmissions.

Education may not always have a positive effect on readmission rates. Investigators who have exclusively focused on the education of patients and their families in the hospital setting have failed to show an independent relationship between educational instructions at discharge and readmission-free survival.[47, 92] In one study, an increase rather than a decrease in rehospitalisation rate was documented after intensive education in the hospital and increased follow up.[93]

Premature discharge

A patient's own assessment seems to be predictive of the need for subsequent readmission. Patients who felt they were discharged too soon were more likely to be readmitted than patients who felt they were ready to be discharged.[36] A researcher who questioned caregivers and patients retrospectively found that both groups identified premature discharge as being a common contributory factor (58%) in unplanned readmission within 28 days of discharge.[17] This assessment was congruent with the patient's general practitioner who judged that in 31% of the cases the patient had been discharged too soon.[17]

No prospective study has been conducted to address the problem of premature discharge. However, Ashton related premature discharge to an increased risk of readmission using a set of criteria to evaluate readiness for discharge.[46] Readiness for discharge was defined as clinical stability, appropriate education of patient and family on medication and diet, and adequate follow-up medical care. Criteria on clinical stability included improvement in signs and symptoms; stable weight; and normal temperature, blood urea nitrogen, serum creatinine level, serum digoxin level, and prothrombin time.[46]

Another important criterion for discharge is the stability of cardiac medication for the preceding 24 hours. Reed and colleagues found that any medication change in the 48 hours prior to discharge was a risk factor for readmission in an older medically ill population.[94] Proper discharge planning by physicians, nurses, and other members of the health-care team is important to facilitate the patient's transition from the hospital to the home environment. In some cases, patients and families need emotional support to decrease their anxiety.[41, 42] For elderly people it may be necessary to make specific arrangements for additional support, such as assistance in obtaining prescribed medication or transportation to doctor's appointments. Elderly patients, who often have an inadequate support system, require more assistance after discharge for a longer period than the general population.[95] Research suggests that comprehensive discharge planning for the hospitalised elderly results in a lower readmission rate and fewer total days of rehospitalisation when clinical nurse specialists combine it with follow-up.[96] Early consultation with social services to facilitate discharge planning is also effective in reducing readmission rates.[62]

Lack of follow-up and inadequate continuity of care

Most patients are discharged without adequate arrangements for assistance from community agencies or home health services, and without adequate rehabilitation.[14, 15, 20] An early study found that almost 40% of heart failure patients discharged directly home were readmitted to hospital within 6 months compared with 20% of those discharged to a secondary facility (skilled nursing facility, rehabilitation centre, or chronic care hospital).[9] The authors reported that the patient with complex problems who is sent directly home appears to be at considerably greater risk of hospital readmission. Similar results were found after controlling for health and socioeconomic factors: those returned to the community for care at home were more likely to be readmitted than those discharged to an institution.[97]

In a general older population, seniors who lived in an institutional setting had a lower risk of readmission than seniors living in their own home.[98] However, the mechanism for the differences in hospital readmissions is not clear. It may be the result of more intensive monitoring by staff in the institutional setting.

Planning for social and environmental support has to be a part of hospital discharge planning. Some experts recommend that a qualified individual – for example, an advanced practice nurse (APN) who is a clinical nurse specialist or nurse practitioner – designs and co-ordinates the discharge plan.[96, 99] To adequately plan the discharge of an older patient, the APN must be knowledgeable about care of the elderly and nursing care for patients with heart failure. An important function of the APN is to provide education and anticipatory guidance for these patients.[96, 100] In addition, the need for centres specialised in the management of patients with heart failure is stressed in the literature.[101]

Data from most studies suggest that heart failure patients who receive appropriate follow-up care have lower hospital readmissions, fewer visits to the emergency room, and lower costs. Different types of follow-up can be considered: mailed reminders of appointments, follow-up by telephone calls to monitor the patient's progress and answer questions, or home visits. Patients in an early study of group education and counselling sessions for heart failure patients had higher levels of knowledge and decreased readmission rates.[102] Home monitoring by a telemedicine system in which daily weight and symptoms are assessed and interpreted by a nurse has been described but awaits experimental testing.[103]

Risk scores for readmission

Several authors have tried to design methods to identify individuals who are at high risk for hospital admission. These risk scores or risk models are often derived from information from administrative data sources, and do not include data on patient compliance, social support, psychosocial status, or participation in care management programmes.

In Table 2.1 a risk model proposed by Chin and Goldman is presented.[21] They developed this model for patients with heart failure and found that both clinical and social factors are important in predicting clinical decline (i.e. readmission or death). The model identified some patients at an especially high risk for readmission or death, but a low-risk group could not be identified. Another model was developed by Philbin and DiSalvo,[23] who identified a method to segregate patients into different risk categories for readmission (Table 2.2). They found that the observed readmission rates within 1 year ranged from 9.8% in patients with risk scores of 0–3 to 45.4% for patients with scores greater than 11 points. This model combines different clinical and demographic factors. However, overall it is still difficult to find a model that perfectly predicts resource utilisation.

Table 2.1 Risk score for readmission or death within 60 days in patients with heart failure.

Marital status	
Single	2 points
Comorbidity (Charlson comorbidity index)	
1	1 point
2	2 points
3	3 points
4 and higher	4 points
Initial systolic blood pressure	
< 101 mmHg	3 points
ECG	
No ST-T wave changes*	2 points

Risk score	Readmission or death/number of patients	Percentage readmitted or dead within 60 days (95% CI)
0–1	0 /17	0 (0–20)
2–5	34/144	24 (17–31)
6–7	30/71	42 (31–55)
>7	18/25	72 (51–88)

Adapted from Chin & Goldman.[21]
*On initial electrocardiogram, neither known to be old nor attributable to digoxin.

Table 2.2 Calculation of simple risk score for readmission in a heart failure patient.

	Points
Baseline value	*4*
For each of the following present:	*Add 1 point*
Black race	
Medicare insurance[a]	
Medicaid insurance[a]	
Home health care services after discharge	
Ischaemic heart diseases	
Valvular heart disease	
Diabetes mellitus	
Renal disease	
Chronic lung disease	
Idiopathic cardiomyopathy	
Prior cardiac surgery	
Use of telemetry during index hospitalisation	
For each of the following present:	*Subtract 1 point*
Treatment in a rural hospital	
Discharge to skilled nursing facility	
Echocardiogram performed during index hospitalisation	
Cardiac catheterisation performed during index hospitalisation	
Range of possible scores	*0–15*

*Indicates primary insurance, therefore a patient may be given only one point for either Medicare or Medicaid insurance.
Adapted from Philbin and DiSalvo[34]

Conclusion

Rehospitalisation occurs frequently in the heart failure population. Many readmissions are related to patient-related and provider-related factors. Patient characteristics, provider preparation, and processes of care may be used to estimate the risk of hospital readmission for heart failure. Several factors such as demographic and clinical factors cannot be changed. Others, such as factors related to inadequate diagnosis and treatment, can be modified to reduce hospital readmissions.

References

1   Ho KK, Pinsky JL, Kannel WB, Levy D. The epidemiology of heart failure: the Framingham study. *J Am Coll Cardiol* 1993; **22**: 6A–13A.

2   Gillum RF. Epidemiology of heart failure in the United States [editorial]. *Am Heart J* 1993; **126**: 1042–7.
3   Cowie MR, Mosterd A, Wood DA *et al*. The epidemiology of heart failure. Eur Heart J 1997; **18**: 209–25.
4   Mosterd A. *Epidemiology of heart failure*. Doctoral thesis, Erasmus University of Rotterdam, 1997.
5   Hoes AW, Mosterd A, Grobbee DE. An epidemic of heart failure? *Eur Heart J* 1998; **19**(suppl. L): 2–10.
6   McMurray JJV, Petrie MC, Murdoch DR, Davie AP. Clinical epidemiology of heart failure: public and private health burden. *Eur Heart J* 1998; **19**(suppl. P): 9–16.
7   Fleg JL. CHF: reflections on current management of the older patient. Geriatrics 1986; **41**: 971–81.
8   Bonneux L, Barendrecht JJ, Meeter K, Bonsel GJ, van der Maas PJ. Estimating clinical morbidity due to ischaemic heart disease and congestive heart failure: the future rise of heart failure. *Am J Publ Health* 1994; **84**: 20–8.
9   Gooding J, Jette AM. Hospital readmissions among the elderly. *J Am Geriatr Soc* 1985: **33**: 595–601.
10 Vinson JM, Rich MW, Sperry JC. Early readmission of elderly patients with congestive heart failure. *J Am Geriatr Soc* 1990; **38**: 1290–5.
11 Ghali JK, Kadakia S, Cooper R, Ferlinz J. Precipitating factors leading to decompensation of heart failure. *Arch Intern Med* 1988; **148**: 2013–17.
12 Edep ME, Shah NB, Tateo IM, Massie BM. Differences between primary care physicians and cardiologists in management of congestive heart failure: relation to practice guidelines. *J Am Coll Cardiol* 1997; **30**: 518–26.
13 Tavazzi L. Objectives of guidelines on heart failure. *Eur Heart J* 1998; **19**(suppl L):33–5.
14 Nikolaus T, Specht-Leible N, Krusse W, Oster P, Schlierf G. The early rehospitalization of elderly patients; causes and prevention. *Dtsch Med Wschr* 1992; **117**: 403–7.
15 Graham H, Livesley B. Can readmissions to a geriatric medical unit be prevented? *Lancet* 1983; **1**: 404–6.
16 Michalsen A, Konig G, Thimme W. Preventable causative factors leading to hospital admission with decompensated heart failure. *Heart* 1998; **80**: 437–41.
17 Andrews K. Relevance of readmission of elderly patients discharged from a geriatric unit. *J Am Geriatr Soc* 1986; **34**: 15–21.
18 Fethke CL, Smith IM, Johnson N. Risk factors affecting readmission of the elderly into the health care system. *Med Care* 1986; **24**: 429–37.
19 Anderson GF, Steinberg EP. Hospital readmissions in the Medicare population. *N Engl J Med* 1984; **311**: 1349–53.
20 Victor CR, Vetter NJ. The early readmission of the elderly to the hospital. *Age Aging* 1985; **14**: 37–42.
21 Chin MH, Goldman L. Correlates of early hospital readmission or death in patients with congestive heart failure. *Am J Cardiol* 1997; **79**:1640–4.
22 Krumholz HM, Parent EM, Tu N *et al*. Readmission after hospitalisation for congestive heart failure among Medicare beneficiaries. *Arch Intern Med* 1997; **157**: 99–104.
23 Philbin EF, DiSalvo TG. Prediction of hospital readmission for heart failure: development of a simple risk score based on administrative data. *J Am Coll Cardiol* 1999; **33**:1560–6.
24 Boult C, Dowd B, McCaffrey D, Boult L, Hernandez R, Krulewitch H. Screening elders for risk of hospital admission. *J Am Geriatr Soc* 1993; **41**: 811–17.
25 McCusker J, Bellavance F, Cardin S, Trepanier S, Verdon J, Ardman O. Detection of older people at increased risk of adverse health outcomes after an emergency visit: the ISAR screening tool. *J Am Geriatr Soc* 1999; **47**: 1229–37.
26 Johnson MR. Heart failure in women: a special approach? *J Heart Lung Transplant* 1994; **13**: S130.
27 Moser DK. Heart failure in women. *Crit Care Nurs Clin of North Am* 1997; **9**: 511–19.
28 Philbin EF, DiSalvo TG. Influence of race and gender on care process, resource use, and hospital base outcomes in congestive heart failure. *Am J Cardiol* 1998; **82**: 76–81.
29 Pernekil R, Vinson JM, Shah AS, Beckham V, Wittenberg C, Rich MW. Course and prognosis on patients > 70 years of age with congestive heart failure and normal versus abnormal left ventricular ejection fraction. *Am J Cardiol* 1997; **79**: 216–19.

30 Alexander M, Grumbach K, Remy L, Rowell R, Massie BM. Congestive heart failure hospitalizations and survival in California: patterns according to race/ethnicity. *Am Heart J* 1999; **137**: 919–27.

31 Bindman AB, Grumbach K, Osmond D *et al.* Preventable hospitalisations and access to health care. *JAMA* 1995; **274**: 305–11.

32 Kahn KL, Pearson ML, Harrison ER *et al.* Health care for black and poor hospitalized Medicare patients. *JAMA* 1994; **271**: 1169–74.

33 Burns R, Nichols LO. Factors predicting readmission of older general medicine patients. *J Gen Intern Med* 1991; **6**: 389–93.

34 Philbin EF, DiSalvo TG. Managed care for congestive heart failure: influence of payer status on process of care, resource utilization, and short term outcomes. *Am Heart J* 1998; **136**: 553–61.

35 Krumholz HM, Butler J, Miller J *et al.* Prognostic importance of emotional support for elderly patients hospitalized with heart failure. *Circulation* 1998; **97**: 958–64.

36 Williams EL, Fitton F. Factors affecting early unplanned readmission of elderly patients to hospital. *Br Med J* 1988; **297**: 784–7.

37 Burke LE, Dunbar-Jacob J. Adherence to medication, diet, and activity recommendations: from assessment to maintenance. *J Cardiovasc Nurs* 1995; **9**: 62–79.

38 Doherty WJ, Schrott HG, Metcalf L, Iasiello-Vailas L. Effect of spouse support and health beliefs on medication adherence. *J Fam Pract* 1983; **17**: 834–41.

39 Hubbard P, Muhlenkamp AF, Brown N. The relationship between social support and self-care practices. *Nurs Res* 1984; **33**: 266–70.

40 Rich MW, Gray DB, Beckham V, Wittenberg C, Luther P. Effect of a multidisciplinary intervention on medication compliance in elderly patients with congestive heart failure. *Am Med J* 1996; **101**: 270–6.

41 Karmilovich SE. Burden and stress associated with spousal caregiving for individuals with heart failure. *Prog Cardiovasc Nurs* 1994; **9**: 33–8.

42 Doering LV, Dracup K, Tullman D *et al.* What predicts the emotional health of spouses of advanced heart failure patients? *Circulation* 1998 (suppl. I): 64.

43 Harjai KJ, Nunez E, Turgut T *et al.* The independent effects of left ventricular ejection fraction on short-term outcomes and resource utilization following hospitalization for heart failure. *Clin Cardiol* 1999; **22**:184–90.

44 McGrae McDermott M, Feinglass J, Lee PI *et al.* Systolic function, readmission rates, and survival among consecutively hospitalized patients with congestive heart failure. *Am Heart J* 1997; **134**: 728–36.

45 Philbin EF, Rocco TA. Use of angiotensin-converting enzyme inhibitors in heart failure with preserved left ventricular systolic function. *Am Heart J* 1997; **134**: 188–95.

46 Ashton CM, Kuykendall DH, Johnson ML, Wray NP, Wu L. The association between the quality of inpatient care and early readmission. *Ann Int Med* 1995; **122**: 415–21.

47 Jaarsma T, Halfens R, Huijer Abu-Saad H *et al.* Effects of education and support on self-care and resource utilization in patients with heart failure. *Eur Heart J* 1999; **20**: 673–82.

48 Young JB. Contemporary management of patients with heart failure. *Med Clin North Am* 1995; **79**: 1171–90.

49 Philbin EF, Santella RN, Rocco TA. Angiotensin-converting enzyme inhibitor use in older patients with heart failure and renal dysfunction. *J Am Geriatr Soc* 1999; **47**: 302–8.

50 Bittner V, Weiner DH, Yusuf S *et al.* Prediction of mortality and morbidity with a 6-minute walk test in patients with left ventricular dysfunction. *JAMA* 1993; **270**: 1702–7.

51 Belardinelli R, Georgiou D, Cianci G, Purcaro A. Randomized, controlled trial of long-term moderate exercise training in chronic heart failure. *Circulation* 1999; **99**: 1173–82.

52 Freedland KE, Carney RM, Rich MW *et al.* Depression in elderly patients with heart failure. *J Geriatr Psych* 1991; **24**: 59–71.

53 Steinhart MJ. Depression and chronic fatigue in the patient with heart disease. *Prim Care* 1991; **18**: 309–25.

54 Rengo F, Acafora D, Trojano L, Furgi G. Congestive heart failure and cognitive impairment in the elderly. *Arch Gerontol Geriatr* 1995; **20**: 63–8.

55 Koenig HG. Depression in hospitalized older patients with congestive heart failure. *Gen Hosp Psych* 1998; **20**: 29–43.

56 Davidson F, Haghfelt T, Gram LF. Adverse drug reactions and drug noncompliance as primary causes of admission to a cardiology department. *Eur J Clin Pharm* 1988; **34**: 83–6.

57 Monane M, Bohn RL, Gurwitz JH, Glynn RJ, Avorn J. Noncompliance with congestive heart failure therapy in the elderly. *Arch Int Med* 1994; **154**: 433–7.

58 Bertel O. The influence of patient information, compliance and medical regimen on the prognosis of patients with chronic heart failure [German]. Herz 1991; **16**: 294–7.

59 Kostam M, Dracup K, Baker D *et al. Heart failure: evaluation and care of patients with left ventricular systolic dysfunction.* Clinical Practice Guideline No. 11. AHCPR Publication No. 94-0612. Rockville, MD: Agency for Health Care Policy and Research, Public Health Service, US Department of Health and Human Services, June 1994.

60 Rich MW, Vinson JM, Sperry JC *et al.* Prevention of readmission in elderly patients with congestive heart failure. *J Gen Intern Med* 1993; **8**: 585–90.

61 Opasich C, Febo O, Riccardi PG *et al.* Concommitant factors of decompensation in chronic heart failure. Am J Cardiol 1996; **78**: 354–7.

62 Rich MW, Beckham V, Wittenberg C, Leven CL, Freedland KE, Carney RM. A multidisciplinary intervention to prevent the readmission of elderly patients with congestive heart failure. *N Engl J Med* 1995; **333**: 1190–5.

63 Struthers AD. Emerging issues on the role of angiotensin-converting enzyme inhibition in the treatment of cardiac failure. Clin Cardiol 1996; **19**(suppl. I): 2–4.

64 Wagdi P, Vuilliomenet A, Kaufmann U, Richter M, Bertel O. Inadequate treatment compliance, patient information and drug prescription as causes for emergency hospitalisation of patients with chronic heart failure. *Schweiz Med Wschr* 1993: **123**: 108–12.

65 Cline CMJ, Bjorck-Linne A, Israelsson BYA, Willenheimer RB, Erhardt LR. Non-compliance and knowledge of prescribed medication in elderly patients with heart failure. *Eur J Heart Fail* 1999; **1**: 145–51.

66 Bushnell FK. Self-care teaching for congestive heart failure patients. *J Geront Nurs* 1992; **18**(10): 27–32.

67 Sulzbach-Hoke LM, Kagan SH, Craig K. Weighing behaviour and symptom distress of clinic patients with CHF. *Med Surg Nurs* 1997; **6**: 288–93.

68 Berkman B, Dumas S, Gastfriend J, Poplawski J, Southworth M. Predicting hospital readmission of elderly cardiac patients. *Health Soc Work* 1987; **12**: 221–8.

69 Philbin EF, Weil HFXC, Erb TA, Jenkins PL. Cardiology or primary care for heart failure in the community setting. *Chest* 1999; **116**: 346–54.

70 Reis SE, Holubkov R, Edmundowics D. Treatment of patients admitted to the hospital with congestive heart failure: specialty-related disparities in practice patterns and outcomes. *J Am Coll Cardiol* 1997; **30**: 733–8.

71 Weissman JS, Ayanian JZ, Chasan-Taber S, Sherwood MJ, Roth C, Epstein AM. Hospital readmissions and quality of care. Med Care 1999; **37**: 490-501.

72 Fonarov GC, Stevenson LW, Walden JA *et al.* Impact of a comprehensive heart failure management program on hospital readmission and functional status of patients with advanced heart failure. *J Am Coll Cardiol* 1997; **30**: 725–32.

73 Clarke KW, Gray D, Hampton JR. Evidence of inadequate investigation and treatment of patients with heart failure. *Br Heart J* 1994; **71**: 584–7.

74 Hillis GS, Trent RJ, Winton P, *et al.* Angiotensin-converting enzyme inhibitors in the management of cardiac failure: are we ignoring the evidence? *Quart J Med* 1996; **89**: 145–50.

75 McMurray JJV. Failure to practice evidence based medicine: why do physicians not treat patients with heart failure with angiotensin-converting enzyme inhibitors? *Eur Heart J* 1999 (suppl. L); **20**: 15–22.

76 Forman DE, Chander RB, Lapane KL, Shah P, Stoukides J. Evaluating the use of angiotensin-coverting enzyme inhibitors of older nursing home residents with chronic heart failure. *J Am Geriatr Soc* 1998; **46**: 1550–4.

77 Cleland JGF. Health economic consequences of the pharmacological treatment of heart failure. *Eur Heart J* 1998; **19**(suppl. P): 32–9.

78 Garg R, Yusuf S. Overview of randomized trials of angiotensin converting enzyme inhibition on mortality and morbidity in patients with heart failure. *JAMA* 1995; **273**: 1450–6.

79 Luzier AB, Forrest A, Adelman M, Hawari FI, Schentag JJ, Izzo JL. Impact of angiotensin-converting enzyme inhibitor underdosing on rehospitalization rates in congestive heart failure. *Am J Cardiol* 1998; **82**: 465-69.

80 Pfeffer MA, Braunwald E, Moye LA *et al*. Effect of captopril on mortality and morbidity in patients with left ventricular dysfunction after myocardial infarction. *N Engl J Med* 1992; **327**: 669–77.

81 Kruse W. Early readmission of elderly patients with congestive heart failure. *J Am Geriatr Soc* 1991; **39**: 1045–6.

82 Bergman U, Wiholm BE. Drug-related problems causing admission to a medical clinic. *Eur J Clin Pharm* 1981; **20**: 193–200.

83 Dracup K, Baker DW, Dunbar SB *et al*. Management of heart failure: counselling, education and lifestyle modifications. *JAMA* 1994; **272**: 1442–6.

84 Marcantonio ER, McKean S, Goldfinger M, Kleefield S, Yurkofsky M, Brennan TA. Factors associated with unplanned hospital readmission among patients 65 years of age and older in a Medicare managed care plan. *Am Med J* 1999; **107**: 13–17.

85 Stewart S, Pearson S, Horowitz JD. Effects of a home-based intervention among patients with congestive heart failure discharged from acute hospital care. *Arch Intern Med* 1998; **158**: 1067–72.

86 Ashby BSH. *Home teaching: effect on compliance, hospital readmissions and days of rehospitalization for patients with chronic congestive heart failure*. Doctoral dissertation. Richmond: Virginia Commonwealth University, 1988.

87 Weinberger M, Smith DM, Katz BP, Moore PS. The cost-effectiveness of intensive postdischarge care. *Med Care* 1988; **11**: 1092–101.

88 West JA, Miller NH, Parker KM *et al*. A comprehensive management system for heart failure improves clinical outcomes and reduces medical resource utilization. *Am J Cardiol* 1997; **79**: 58–63.

89 Shah NB, Der E, Ruggerio C, Heidenreich PA, Massie BM. Prevention of hospitalization for heart failure with an interactive home monitoring program. *Am Heart J* 1998; **135**: 373–8.

90 Ekman I, Andersson B, Ehnfors M, Matejka G, Persson B, Fagerberg B. Feasibility of a nurse-monitored, outpatient-care programme for elderly patients with moderate-to-severe, chronic heart failure. *Eur Heart J* 1998; **19**: 1254–60.

91 Cline CMJ, Israelsson BYA, Willenheimer RB, Broms K, Erhardt LR. Cost effective management programme for heart failure reduces hospitalization. *Heart* 1998; **80**: 442–6.

92 McGrae McDermott M, Lee P, Mehta S, Gheorgiade M. Patterns of angiotensin converting enzyme inhibitors prescriptions, educational interventions and outcomes among hospitalized patients with heart failure. *Clin Cardiol* 1998; **21**: 261–8.

93 Weinberger M, Oddone EZ, Henderson WG. Does increased access to primary care reduce hospital readmissions? *N Engl J Med* 1996; **334**: 1441–7.

94 Reed RL, Pearlman RA, Buchner DM. Risk factors for early unplanned hospital readmission in the elderly. *J Gen Intern Med* 1991; **6**: 223–8.

95 Johnson H, Fethke C. Postdischarge outcomes and care planning for the hospitalized elderly. In: McCleland E, Kelly K, Buckwater KC, eds. *Continuity of care: advancing the concept of discharge planning*. Orlando: Grune & Stratton, 1985.

96 Naylor MD, Brooten D, Campbell R *et al*. Comprehensive discharge planning and home-follow-up of hospitalized elders. *JAMA* 1999; **281**: 613–20.

97 Lockerly SA, Dunkle RE, Kart C, Coulton C. Factors contributing to the early rehospitalization of elderly people. *Health Soc Work* 1994; **19**: 182–91.

98 Chu LW, Pei CKW. Risk factors for early emergency hospital readmission in elderly medical patients. *Gerontology* 1999; **45**: 220–6.

99 Hendriksen C, Lund E, Stromgard E. Consequences of assessment and intervention among elderly people: a three-year randomized controlled trial. *Br Med J* 1984; **289**: 1522–4.

100 Kegel LM. Advanced practice nurses can refine the management of heart failure. *Clin Nurse Spec* 1995; **9**: 76–81.

101 Smith LE, Fabbri SA, Pai R, Ferry D, Heywood JT. Symptomatic improvement and reduced hospitalization for patients attending a cardiomyopathy clinic. *Clin Cardiol* 1997; **20**: 949–54.

102 Rosenberg SG. Patient education leads to better care for heart patients. *HSMHA Health Reports* 1971; **86**: 793–802.

103 Mancini D, Cordisco MA, Beniaminovits A, Prince M. Use of telemedical monitoring to decrease rate of hospitalization in patients with severe heart failure. *Circulation* 1998 (suppl. I): 483.

3: Specialist nurse intervention in chronic heart failure: a critical review

SIMON STEWART, LYNDA BLUE

As discussed in Chapter 1, chronic heart failure exerts a heavy burden upon both the individual and society overall. It continues to be associated with increasing hospitalisation rates and significant health-care costs,[1, 2] poorer than average health-related quality of life[3] and premature mortality.[4]

A number of pharmacological agents, for example, angiotensin-converting enzyme (ACE) inhibitors,[5] digoxin,[6] and (more recently) β-adrenoceptor blockers[7] and spironolactone,[8] have been shown to markedly ameliorate the debilitating symptoms commonly associated with this complex syndrome and, in some cases, improve survival. However, the clinical trial environment differs from "usual" clinical practice because the patient is normally managed in a closely monitored environment and receives higher doses of pharmacological agents.

Moreover, despite the apparent advantage of being managed within a clinical trial environment, for those individuals fortunate enough to be randomised to the most effective arm of pharmacological treatment, residual morbidity and mortality rates remain high. For example, in the "treatment" arm of the SOLVD trial, 35% of patients in the enalapril group died within 3.5 years of follow-up, 46% were admitted to hospital with worsening heart failure, and 69% were admitted to hospital for any reason.[9]

This chapter provides a critical overview of the evidence supporting the use of specialist nurse-led interventions in the management of heart failure following acute hospitalisation.

The role of adjunctive, non-pharmacological interventions in heart failure

In lieu of a major advance in the pharmacological management of heart failure, there is an increasing need to develop adjunctive, non-pharmacological strategies that optimise the management of older patients with heart failure.[10–12] Research groups from a number of developed countries have taken up this challenge and applied a similar process in developing effective non-pharmacological strategies. This process includes:

- identifying the subset of "high risk" chronic heart failure patients who experience relatively poorer health outcomes overall, and determining their clinical and demographic characteristics
- identifying the deficiencies in the local health-care system that contribute to these poor health outcomes.
- designing and testing innovative interventions that simultaneously target high-risk individuals and the preventable factors (relating to both the individual and their overall health-care management) that lead to poor health outcomes
- undertaking a properly powered, randomised, controlled study of the intervention to determine whether it is associated with a significant reduction in health-care utilisation (particularly hospital admissions) and improved quality of life relative to that of usual care.

Considering the disproportionate burden of hospital costs to the overall expenditure related to management of chronic heart failure,[2] any intervention that significantly reduces this component of health-care utilisation is likely to be cost-effective.[13]

Identifying high-risk patients

As discussed in Chapter 2, many studies have specifically examined the clinical and demographic characteristics and health outcomes of patients who require hospital-based care for chronic heart failure.[14–19] These studies are undoubtedly biased in that such patients are more likely to have severe heart failure and receive more extensive and intensive specialist care (whether it be on an inpatient or outpatient basis) than the majority of heart failure patients. However, it is on this basis that they are most useful in identifying the most problematic or high-risk patients. These patients have already "revealed" themselves as relatively higher in risk than the majority of patients who avoid prolonged contact with large health-care institutions, and they are differentiated on the basis of their response or non-responsiveness to what should be optimal and intensive treatment. Many studies include both patients specifically hospitalised for heart failure, and those in whom this condition was an associated diagnosis. In

33

some cases the distinction might be nebulous (for example, concurrent pneumonia). Although these studies vary in location, inclusion criteria, size of cohort, and duration of follow-up, the profile and outcomes of these hospitalised patients highlight a number of factors and issues relevant to identifying high-risk individuals.

Overall, it is clear that relatively unselected heart failure patients bear little resemblance (both in terms of baseline demographic and clinical characteristics and subsequent health outcomes) to the majority of those participating in clinical trials. This phenomenon is not confined to heart failure but is also evident in the context of myocardial infarction.[20] The most obvious differences between these conditions are the age of patients and the inherent sex imbalance among clinical trial patients.[21, 22] In general, high-risk patients with chronic heart failure can be identified on the following basis:

- advanced age
- the presence of comorbidity likely to complicate treatment and contribute to higher morbidity and mortality rates
- a history of heart failure-related hospitalisation.

Factors likely to contribute to frequent hospitalisation

The apparent inability of many individuals to gain the maximal clinical benefit from therapy of proven effectiveness is a vexing problem. It is not, however, surprising, considering the complex interaction between the individual, the treatment, and the many components of the health-care system concerned. Anything that interrupts or hinders what should be a harmonious and productive interaction between the patient and the health-care system has the potential to cause lack of symptomatic control, unplanned hospitalisation, and even premature death. Whilst inherently high-risk patients would benefit most from appropriate and consistent treatment, they are, unfortunately, at greatest risk from factors that commonly precipitate suboptimal treatment. Their frequent inability to tolerate even minor fluctuations in their cardiac function leaves them vulnerable to frequent and recurrent episodes of acute heart failure. They are therefore at risk of both frequent hospitalisation for heart failure and other concurrent disease states. For example, the circumstance of concomitant moderate impairment of renal function, particularly due to renovascular disease, is of particular importance in this regard.[23] This problem is more likely to be present in elderly patients,[24] and presents both an incremental hazard to the successful use of ACE inhibitors as well as a basis for increased risk of digitalis toxicity. Whilst such patients tend to be excluded from clinical trials in heart failure, their considerable prevalence in hospitalised cohorts presents a therapeutic dilemma (especially in respect to balancing the risks of drug toxicity versus undertreatment) with no obvious solution.

As discussed in greater detail in Chapter 2, there are many preventable and often interrelated factors contributing to poorer health outcomes among heart failure patients which can be addressed through non-pharmacological means. These potentially modifiable factors can be summarised as follows:

- inadequate or inappropriate pharmacotherapy
- non-compliance with prescribed treatment
- adverse effects of prescribed treatment
- inadequate knowledge of chronic heart failure and prescribed treatment
- inadequate follow-up or suboptimal use of available health care
- poor social support
- early clinical deterioration.

Studies examining strategies to reduce hospital readmissions among the chronically ill

A number of non-pharmacological strategies have been developed to address the aforementioned factors and thereby reduce the frequency of hospitalisation among chronically ill patients. Such strategies often include incremental attention to one or more of the following:

- discharge planning
- comprehensive "geriatric assessment"
- access to primary care services
- access to specialised outpatient clinics
- home-based follow-up.

Table 3.1 summarises the major randomised, controlled trials of non-pharmacological interventions targeting the chronically ill, reported between 1988 and 1999. In response to the growing burden of heart failure, an increasing number of these studies are either specifically designed for, or include a high proportion of, patients with chronic heart failure. The following section represents a more detailed description of those studies involving a major proportion of patients with chronic heart failure.

The evidence in favour of specialist nurse-led strategies

Randomised, controlled studies

To date there have been eight "scientifically sound" (appropriately powered and with complete follow-up), randomised, controlled studies of non-pharmacological interventions designed to reduce hospital use in

35

Table 3.1 Randomised, controlled studies examining the effects of strategies designed to limit hospital readmission among the chronically ill.

Reference	Study cohort	Study intervention	Major end-points	Results	Comments
Stewart, et al. 1999[25] Australia	**200** CHF patients aged (55 yr from a university hospital who were discharged home	Multidisciplinary, home-based intervention with at least one home visit by a cardiac nurse	Frequency of unplanned readmissions plus out-of-hospital deaths within 6 months.	Usual-care patients had more (129 v 77) primary events (p= 0.02) and more intervention patients remained event-free (38 vs 51; p= 0.04) at 6 months	This is the first study to show that this type of intervention is associated with both prolonged event-free survival and fewer readmissions
Naylor, et al. 1999[26] USA	**363** chronically ill patients (mean age 75 yr) from a university hospital, discharged home	Comprehensive discharge planning and a home-based follow-up protocol	Hospital readmissions plus event-free survival within 24 weeks.	Fewer study patients were readmitted (20% v 37%: p< 0.01) and they had more event-free survival (p< 0.001).	Only 70% of intervention and 73% of usual-care patients completed this study
Jaarsma, et al. 1999[27] Netherlands	**179** CHF patients from a university hospital, discharged home	A supportive education program in the hospital and home promoting self-care behaviour	Self-care behaviour and health-care utilisation within 9 months.	The intervention increased self-care behaviour. There were strong associated trends towards fewer patients readmitted and fewer days of admission	This singular strategy was beneficial overall, although none of the health-care utilisation end-points reached statistical significance
Nikolaus et al. 1999[28] Germany	**545** patients with acute illness admitted from home to a university-affiliated geriatric hospital	Comprehensive geriatric assessment alone or this plus additional home-based assessment	Survival, readmission and functional status within 12 months.	There was no difference in survival or acute care readmissions but the intervention was associated with fewer days of readmission	This was an elderly cohort with much more prolonged index hospitalisation compared to other studies of its type
Cline, et al. 1998[29] Sweden	**190** CHF patients aged 65–84 yr, admitted to a university-affiliated hospital and discharged home	In-hospital counselling, plus incremental follow-up at a nurse-led, heart failure-specific outpatient clinic	Time to readmission, duration of hospital stay and health-care costs within 12 months.	Mean time to first admission was prolonged in study patients (p< 0.05). There were no significant differences in survival, hospital stay, and health-care costs at 1yr	Patients were not specifically selected on the basis of risk. However, there were strong trends in favour of study patients in all outcomes studied
Stewart, et al. 1998[30] Australia	**762** chronically ill patients admitted to a university-affiliated hospital and discharged home	In-hospital counselling followed by a single home visit by a nurse and pharmacist	Frequency of unplanned readmissions plus out-of-hospital deaths within 6 months.	Intervention patients had fewer primary events (155 v 155, p< 0.001) and fewer all-cause deaths (12 v 29, p< 0.01)	While this intervention was effective overall, the greatest benefit occurred in the subset of 98 patients with CHF (both at 6 and 18 months)
Siu, et al. 1996[31] USA	**354** patients aged > 65yr admitted to medical and surgical units of a university-affiliated hospital and discharged home	Home visits at 1–3 days post discharge and 3 more visits thereafter as part of geriatric assessment	Survival, frequency of readmissions and nursing home admission within 2 months	No differences between groups were detected as regards mortality, hospital readmission, nursing home placements, and quality of life	Patients were not selected on the basis of risk. Study follow-up was limited to 60 days
Weinberger, et al. 1996[32] USA	**1396** veterans (men) admitted to 9 Veterans Affairs Medical Centers with diabetes, chronic obstructive pulmonary disease or CHF	Close follow-up by a nurse and primary care physician for 6 months following discharge using a clinic-based approach	Frequency of hospital admissions and duration of stay within 6 months	Study patients had higher rates of readmission (0.19 vs 0.14 per month p< 0.01) and more days of hospitalisation (10.2 v 8.8: p< 0.05) relative to that of usual care	This is the only reported trial of an intervention designed to reduce hospitalisation in which more hospitalisations in the intervention group were documented
Rich, et al. 1995[33] USA	**282** high risk CHF patients aged > 70yr from the medical units of a university medical center, discharged home	Nurse-directed, multi-disciplinary intervention involving home and clinic visits	Event-free survival, rate of readmission, quality of life, and cost of care within 3 months	Event-free survival favoured study patients (p=0.09). Study patients had fewer readmissions, better quality of life and fewer health-care costs (p< 0.05)	This was the first, properly powered, randomised study of a nurse-led intervention in CHF
Melin, et al. 1995[34] Sweden	**249** "elderly" patients from medical and surgical units at a county general hospital, discharged home.	Coordinated primary care plus comprehensive in-home assessment and intervention equivalent to 'normal' home care	Mortality, activities of daily living and health-care utilisation within 6 months	There were no differences between groups as regards activities of daily living and survival at 6 months. However, study patients had reduced institutional stays and associated costs	Patients were selected on the basis of risk for increased health-care utilisation. Chronic cardiac illness and more medications at discharge increased risk of death

Study	Patients	Intervention	Outcomes measured	Results	Comments
Fitzgerald, et al. 1994[35] USA	668 patients aged ≥45 yr from medical units at a Veterans Affairs medical center, discharged home	A nurse case-manager arranged clinic follow-up, telephone contact, and provided extra education	Frequency of hospital readmissions and duration of hospital stay within 12 months.	Although patients had more visits to the hospital-based clinic ($p< 0.01$) there were no differences as regards readmissions or duration of hospital stay.	Patients were not selected on the basis of risk. The authors concluded that home visits may be more effective
Naylor, et al. 1994[36] USA	276 patients aged ≥70 years from a university hospital who were either medical or surgical cardiac patients, discharged home.	Incremental discharge planning and telephone contact for 2 weeks post discharge	Duration of index stay, time to first admission, rate of hospitalisation and costs within 3 months.	There were no differences as regards index stay, time to readmission, frequency of readmission, and total costs	Patients were not selected on the basis of risk. Early benefits at 6 weeks post discharge were attenuated by 3 months
Thomas, et al. 1993[37] USA	120 patients aged ≥70 yr from medical and surgical units at a community hospital discharged to either home or long-term care	In-hospital, multifaceted geriatric assessment	Duration of index stay, health-care utilisation and mortality within 6 months.	Significantly fewer deaths and readmissions at 6 months among study patients but no differences in duration of hospital stay at 6 months or survival at 12 months	Patients were not selected on the basis of risk. Data relating to discharge destination are not presented
Evans and Hendricks 1993[38] USA	835 patients aged ≥70 yr from medical and surgical units at a Veterans Affairs Medical Center, discharged to either home or a nursing home	Incremental discharge planning and in-hospital counselling	Health-care utilisation within 9 months.	Despite an early difference in readmission rates at 1 month (24% v 35%; $p< 0.001$) favouring study patients there was no difference at 9 months except reduced days of hospitalisation ($p< 0.001$)	Patients were selected on the basis of risk for increased health-care utilisation. Readmission rates were higher than other reported studies of this type
Winograd, et al. 1993[39] USA	197 patients (men) aged ≥65yr from medical and surgical units at a Veterans Affairs Medical Center, discharged home	Inpatient, multifaceted geriatric consultation.	Activities of daily living, mental status, morale and health-care utilisation within 12 months.	There were no differences between groups at 12 month, except improved mental function among study patients	Patients were not specifically selected on the basis of risk; however, 75% were chronically ill
Rubin, et al. 1992[40] USA	200 patients aged ≥70yr from medical units at an acute care county hospital, discharged to home	Long-term comprehensive geriatric care and multifaceted outpatient care	Health care charges and Medicare costs within 12 months	There was a non-significant reduction in total charges and reimbursement among intervention patients	Post-hoc analysis revealed "fewer hospital readmissions and shorter lengths of stay" among study patients
Hansen, et al. 1992[41] Denmark	344 patients aged ≥75 years from medical and surgical units of a general hospital, discharged home	Visited at one day post-hospitalisation by district nurse and 2 weeks later by a general practitioner	Health care utilisation within 12 months	10/163 trial v 25/181 control patients were admitted to a nursing home ($p< 0.05$). No difference between groups as regards hospital readmission and mortality	Whilst home visits were designed to "identify new and unforeseen problems", patients were not selected on the basis of risk and there were minimal benefits
Smith, et al. 1988[42] USA	1001 patients from medical units of a university-affiliated hospital and discharged to home	Incremental discharge planning and telephone contact designed to increase clinic contacts	Frequency of postdischarge ambulatory contacts and frequency of readmissions with 6 months	Despite a significant increase in clinic-based contacts study patients had similar numbers of unplanned readmissions	The study intervention appeared to have some benefical effects among patients prospectively designated as "high risk"
Townsend, et al. 1988[43] UK	464 "elderly" patients from medical and surgical units at a community hospital, discharged home	Support from care attendants on first day at home and for up to 12hr a week for 2 weeks	Patient "independence", morale and health-care utilisation within 3 months	There were no differences between groups at 3 months; however, at 18 months, study patients had fewer readmissions ($p< 0.05$) and days in hospital ($p< 0.05$)	The authors do not adequately explain why the brief home-support had no initial effects

patients with chronic heart failure discharged from acute hospital care. These studies can be categorised according to the effect of the study intervention on subsequent health-care utilisation.

Negative trials

Perhaps unsurprisingly, considering the inherent bias towards the publication of positive studies, only one negative study of this type has been reported. Weinberger and colleagues described a study in which 1 396 veterans (all men) hospitalised with chronic obstructive pulmonary disease, diabetes, or heart failure were randomised either to usual care or to increased access to primary care nurses and physicians.[32] Patients who received this extra care had a greater number of readmissions to hospital, but were more satisfied with their medical care during 6 months of follow-up. It was postulated at the time that the increased health-care utilisation seen in this group resulted from a combination of greater vigilance in detecting problems and the ability of those detecting such problems (the physicians) to admit patients – thereby lowering admission thresholds.[44] This "clinical cascade" effect represents an important caveat when considering the potential impact of this type of intervention. Although some notable commentators in this field would consider this particular study and its results as having little relevance to more comprehensive, heart failure-specific programmes,[45] we would argue to the contrary. Whilst increased nursing contact with patients is likely to result in more clinical problems being detected, there is also the potential for increased hospitalisation rates if a specialist nurse is empowered to directly admit patients to hospital.

Inconclusive trials

In 1994 Naylor and colleagues described a controlled study of a comprehensive discharge planning protocol implemented by advanced practice nurses. Completed in 1992, this study demonstrated short-term – but not sustained – reductions in readmissions and decreased costs of care for older hospitalised patients with a number medical cardiac conditions (including heart failure) who were managed according to this protocol.[36] More recently, this group has examined the effects of this protocol plus a component of home-based follow-up (a series of home visits by advanced practice nurses). They reported that the intervention was associated with fewer hospital readmissions and days of associated hospitalisation within 24 weeks; although only a small proportion of patients had chronic heart failure and there was significant amount of loss to follow-up (approximately 30%).[26]

More recently, Jaarsma and colleagues examined the effects of a heart failure-specific, home-based educational programme undertaken by a specialist heart failure nurse.[27] This study was specifically undertaken to determine whether a single intervention designed to increase self-care behaviour in patients with chronic heart failure was effective enough to reduce hospital readmissions by a significant margin. Despite an adequate sample size, this study demonstrated that whilst education alone had the potential to reduce hospital readmissions overall, cost-effective thresholds were not reached. For example, during a 9-month follow-up 37% of intervention patients (n = 84) compared with 50% of usual care patients (n = 95) were readmitted to hospital (p = 0.06). Patients exposed to the study intervention also tended to have fewer cardiac-related days of readmission than usual-care patients (427 v 681 days; p = 0.096).

Although the studies described above may appear to provide inconclusive proof of the merits of additional inpatient discharge planning and home-based education following discharge, they are clearly important for a number of reasons. First, they provide a clear indication that they are inherently valuable strategies – even if not associated with a clinically significant reduction in health-care utilisation. Second, when combined with other types of strategies they have the potential to be cost-effective in reducing hospital readmissions.

Positive trials

In the first properly powered and conducted study of its type, Rich and colleagues[33] reported that a nurse-led, multidisciplinary intervention (which involved a component of home visits) had beneficial effects on rates of hospital readmission, quality of life, and cost of care within 90 days of discharge among high-risk patients with chronic heart failure. The intervention consisted of comprehensive education of the patient and family, a prescribed diet, social service consultation and planning for an early discharge, optimisation of pharmacotherapy, and intensive home and clinic-based follow-up with frequent telephone contact. On this basis, the intervention was successful and appeared to slow the typical cycle of recurrent hospitalisation in this type of patient. At 90 days, survival without readmission was achieved in 91 of 142 (64%) intervention patients compared with 75 of 140 (54%) control patients (p = 0.09). There were 94 and 53 readmissions in the control and intervention groups respectively (p = 0.02). Of the total readmissions, 78 (53%) were for heart failure, and there was a disproportionate reduction (56%) of these types of readmissions in the intervention group (24 v 54; p = 0.04). Importantly, fewer intervention group patients had more than one readmission (9 v 23; p = 0.01). These results were associated with significantly better quality of life and reduced health costs among intervention patients.

In 1998, Cline and colleagues also reported the benefits of a clinic-based follow-up of a lower-risk cohort of patients with chronic heart failure.[29] A total of 206 older patients hospitalised with heart failure were randomised to the study intervention or to usual care. The special intervention included an education programme for patients and their families, concentrating on treatment. Guidelines for adjusting treatment in response to sodium and water overload and fluid depletion were also provided. This programme was carried out over two 30-minute visits to the patient in hospital and a 1-hour home visit to the patient and family 2 weeks after discharge. Frequent and easily accessible patient-initiated follow-up was provided in the form of a nurse-run, hospital-based clinic and telephone contact. During 12 months of follow-up, time to first readmission was a third longer in the intervention group (106 v 141 days; p < 0.05). The intervention was also associated with a strong trend towards fewer hospital admissions, fewer days of hospitalisation, and lower cost of care during study follow-up in comparison with those reported by Rich and colleagues.[33] It is likely that type II error prevented the intervention being shown to be significantly better in this regard. The results of this study therefore tend to reinforce the need to select a higher-risk subset of patients in order to target interventions in a cost-efficient manner.

Following post-hoc analyses of a large-scale, randomised, controlled study of chronically ill patients with a mixture of cardiac and non-cardiac disease states,[30] which showed that a nurse-led, multidisciplinary, home-based intervention was most effective in chronic heart failure patients,[46, 47] Stewart and colleagues prospectively examined such an intervention more specifically designed for these patients.[25] Patients with chronic heart failure discharged home following acute hospitalisation were randomised to usual care ($n = 100$) or to multidisciplinary, home-based intervention ($n = 100$). The intervention primarily consisted of a home visit 7–14 days after discharge by a cardiac nurse to identify and address issues likely to result in unplanned hospitalisation. The primary end-point for the study was frequency of unplanned readmission plus out-of-hospital death within 6 months. During 6 months follow-up the primary end-point occurred more frequently in the usual-care group (129 v 77 primary events; p = 0.02). More intervention patients remained event-free (38 v 51; p = 0.04). Overall, there were fewer unplanned readmissions (68 v 118; p = 0.03) and associated days of hospitalisation (460 v 1173; p = 0.02) among patients assigned to the study intervention. Consequently, hospital-based costs for the intervention group tended to be lower than those for usual care (AU $490 300 vs $922 600; p = 0.16). The mean cost of the intervention was AU$350 per patient; other community-based costs were similar for both groups. The frequency distribution of unplanned readmissions was significantly different for the two groups (p = 0.04) with fewer intervention patients (5 v 19) requiring three or more readmissions. In a subgroup of 68 patients, heart failure specific (p = 0.04) and general quality of life scores (p = 0.01) at 3 months were most improved among those assigned to multidisciplinary, home-based intervention. Furthermore, assignment to the study intervention was an independent predictor of survival at 6 months (adjusted relative risk 0.54; p = 0.046).[25]

Two controlled studies, one involving a clinic-based and the other a home-based approach to the management of heart failure, have been completed in New Zealand and Scotland respectively. The researchers themselves describe these studies and their positive effects on health-care utilisation in Chapters 5 and 7 of this book. Overall, the results are consistent with the literature to date and provide incremental support for the use of specialist nurse-led interventions in heart failure.

Non-randomised studies

The results of the randomised studies described above are broadly consistent with those of non-randomised studies of similar strategies targeting older, hospitalised heart failure patients. For example, Kornowski and colleagues reported that an intensive home-based intervention by physicians was associated with reduced hospitalisation rates and improved quality of life in such patients (n = 42).[48] Similarly, West and colleagues reported that an intensive physician-supervised, nurse-mediated, home-based system for heart failure management (the MULTI-FIT programme) was associated with improved functional status and exercise capacity and reduced hospitalisation rates among both previously hospitalised and clinic-managed heart failure patients (n = 51).[49] Fonarow and colleagues also reported favourable effects associated with a comprehensive management programme targeting younger patients awaiting heart transplantation.[50] More recently, Shah and colleagues reported on the preliminary results of a study examining a nurse-led electronic monitoring programme, incorporating a strategy to facilitate patient self-monitoring of their heart failure status and weekly reminder calls by nurses; this programme reduced subsequent hospitalisation among a small cohort (n = 27) of both older and middle-aged patients with chronic heart failure.[51]

Which type of specialist nurse-led intervention is best?

It appears that interventions involving a component of home-based follow-up by a specialist nurse, are more effective than those incorporating clinic-based follow-up. Similarly, a clinic-based approach appears to be more effective than strategies confined to the period of acute hospitalisation (for example, incremental discharge planning).

The results of studies examining the effect of home-based intervention suggest that such programmes have the potential to prolong event-free survival, reduce the number of readmissions within a year of index hospitalisation by approximately 50%, and prolong survival without adversely affecting quality of life. However, simply visiting patients at home and counselling them is obviously not enough,[27] and an interdisciplinary approach is more effective.

These conclusions are largely based upon randomised, controlled studies. A number of historical control studies undertaken in the USA suggest that a clinic-based approach may be more beneficial than home-based intervention. However, such studies should be interpreted with caution as they have an inherent bias in favour of the intervention by counting the qualifying event as an end-point during the historical control period.

Patients unwilling to be managed by a specialist nurse using a home-based approach would certainly benefit from being managed by a specialist nurse-led outpatient clinic. Moreover, excepting the study performed by Rich and colleagues which limited follow-up to 3 months,[33] there is a paucity of studies examining the potential value of the combination of home and clinic-based follow-up – an approach that may prove to be the most effective of all. Furthermore, research is still needed to establish the optimal timing and frequency of interventions that have already proved to be effective. Chapter 9 summarises the essential components of successful specialist nurse-led interventions in heart failure.

Residual issues

Although specialist nurse-led interventions have been shown to be effective in improving health outcomes in chronic heart failure, this is still an evolving field of health care, and a number of important issues remain unresolved:

- What is the future role of this type of intervention given the evolving armoury of pharmacological agents?
- What are the minimum qualifications needed by a specialist nurse in heart failure in order to be effective?
- Who should oversee the role and actions of specialist nurses and how independent should they become?
- What is the best way to integrate a specialist nurse service into the pre-existing health-care structure?
- How do you measure and maintain the quality of this type of intervention?
- Most importantly, who should fund this type of intervention?

Certainly, translating research into practice puts additional pressure on the architects of such interventions to apply only the essential components of their intervention. Chapter 10 describes the type of process required to implement this type of intervention and attempts to address these issues in greater detail.

Conclusions

Specialist nurse-led interventions in heart failure, especially when incorporating a interdisciplinary approach and home visits, are particularly effective in improving health outcomes among heart failure patients. As long as they are adapted to the local health care environment, they represent a cost-effective means of reducing hospital use in patients with chronic heart failure and improving their overall quality of life.

References

1   Haldeman GA, Croft JB, Giles WH, Rashidee A. Hospitalization of patients with heart failure: national hospital discharge survey 1985-1995. *Am Heart J* 1999; **137**: 352–60.
2   McMurray JJ, Petrie MC, Murdoch DR, Davie AP. Clinical epidemiology of heart failure: public and private health burden. *Eur Heart J* 1998; **19**: 9–16.
3   Stewart AL, Greenfield S, Hays RD *et al.* Functional status and well-being of patients with chronic conditions: results from the medical outcomes study. *JAMA* 1989; **262**: 907–13.
4   Ho KKL, Anderson KM, Karmel WB *et al.* Survival after the onset of congestive heart failure in the Framingham Heart Study subjects. Circulation 1993; **88**: 107–15.
5   Swedberg K, Kjekshus J, Snapinn S. Long-term survival in severe heart failure in patients treated with enalapril. Ten year follow-up of CONSENSUS 1. *Eur Heart J* 1999; **2**: 136–39.
6   The Digitalis Investigation Group. The effect of digoxin on mortality and morbidity in patients with heart failure. *N Engl J Med* 1997; **336**: 525–33.
7   MERIT Investigators. Effect of metoprolol CR/XL in chronic heart failure: Metoprolol CR/XL Randomised Intervention Trial in Congestive Heart Failure (Merit-HF). *Lancet* 1999; **353**: 2001–7.
8   Pitt B, Zannad F, Remme WJ *et al.* The effect of spironolactone on morbidity and mortality in patients with severe heart failure. Randomized Aldactone Evaluation Study Investigators. *N Engl J Med* 1999; **341**: 709–17.
9   The SOLVD Investigators. Effect of enalapril on survival in patients with reduced left ventricular ejection fractions and congestive heart failure. *N Engl J Med* 1991; **325**: 293–302.
10 Sharpe N. Heart failure management – a broader view required [editorial]. *Eur Heart J* 1998; **19**: 975.
11 McMurray J, Stewart S. Nurse-led, multidisciplinary intervention in chronic heart failure [editorial]. *Heart* 1998; **80**: 430-1.
12 Krum H. Reducing the burden of chronic heart failure [editorial]. *Med J Aust* 1997; **167**: 61–2.
13 Mark DB. Economics of treating heart failure. *Am J Cardiol* 1997; **80**: 33H-38H.
14 Jaagosild P, Dawson N, Thomas C *et al.* Outcomes of acute exacerbation of severe congestive heart failure. *Arch Intern Med* 1998; **158**: 1081–9.
15 Lowe J, Candlish P, Henry D, Wlodarcyk J, Heller R, Fletcher P. Management and outcomes of congestive heart failure: a prospective study of hospitalised patients. *Med J Aust* 1998; **168**: 115–18.
16 Wolinsky F, Smith D, Stump T, Overhage J, Lubitz R. The sequale of hospitalisation for congestive heart failure among older adults. *J Am Geriatr Soc* 1997; **45**: 558–63.
17 Krumholz HM, Parent EM, Tu N *et al.* Readmission after hospitalisation for congestive heart failure among medicare beneficiaries. *Arch Intern Med* 1997; **157**: 99–104.
18 Ni H, Naumann D, Hershberger R. Managed care and outcomes of hospitalization among elderly patients with congestive heart failure. *Arch Intern Med* 1998; **158**: 1231–6.

19 Blyth F, Lazarus R, Ross D, Price M, Cheuk G, Leeder S. Burden and outcomes of hospitalisation for congestive heart failure. *Med J Aust* 1997; **167**: 67–70.

20 Gurwitz J, Col N, Avorn J. The exclusion of the elderly and women from clinical trials in acute myocardial infarction. *JAMA* 1992; **268**: 1417–22.

21 Cohen-Salal A, Delahaye F, Desnos M, Ermeriau J, Hanania G. Who are the patients hospitalised for heart failure in France today? [abstract] *Eur Heart J* 1998; **19** (suppl.): 248.

22 Petrie MC, Dawson NF, Murdoch DR, Davie AP, McMurray JJ. Failure of women's hearts. *Circulation* 1999; **99**: 2334–41.

23 MacDowall P, Kaira P, O'Donoghue D, Waldek S, Mamtora H, Brown K. Risk of morbidity from renovascular disease in elderly patients with congestive cardiac failure. *Lancet* 1998; **352**: 13–16.

24 Brown A, Cleland J. Influence of concomitant disease on patterns of hospitalization in patients with heart failure discharged from Scottish hospitals in 1995. *Eur Heart J* 1998; **19**: 1063–9.

25 Stewart S, Marley JE, Horowitz JD. Effects of a multidisciplinary, home-based intervention on unplanned readmissions and survival among patients with chronic congestive heart failure: a randomised controlled study. *Lancet* 1999; **354**: 1077–83.

26 Naylor MD, Brooten D, Cambell R *et al.* Comprehensive discharge planning and home follow-up of hospitalized elders: a randomized clinical trial. *JAMA* 1999; **281**: 613–20.

27 Jaarsma T, Halfens R, Huijer Abu-Saad H *et al.* Effects of education and support on self-care and resource utilization in patients with heart failure. *Eur Heart J* 1999; **20**: 673–82.

28 Nikolaus T, Specht-Leible N, Bach M, Oster P, Schlierf G. A randomized trial of comprehensive geriatric assessment and home intervention in the care of hospitalized patients. *Age Aging* 1999; **28**: 543–50.

29 Cline C, Israelsson B, Willenheimer R *et al.* A cost effective management programme for heart failure reduces hospitalisation. *Heart* 1998; **80**: 442–6.

30 Stewart S, Pearson S, Luke CG, Horowitz JD. Effects of a home based intervention on unplanned readmissions and out-of-hospital deaths. *J Am Geriatr Soc* 1998; **46**: 174–80.

31 Siu AL, Kravitz RL, Keeler E *et al.* Postdischarge geriatric assessment of hospitalized frail elderly patients. *Arch Intern Med* 1996; **156**: 76–81.

32 Weinberger M, Oddone EZ, Henderson WG. Does increased access to primary care reduce hospital readmissions? *N Engl J Med* 1996; **334**: 1441–7.

33 Rich MW, Beckham V, Wittenberg C, Leven CL, Freedland KE, Carney RM. A multidisciplinary intervention to prevent the readmission of elderly patients with congestive heart failure. *N Engl J Med* 1995; **333**: 1190–5.

34 Melin AL, Wieland D, Harker JO, Bygren LO. Health outcomes of post-hospital in-home team care: second Swedish trial. *J Am Geriatr Soc* 1995; **43**: 301–7.

35 Fitzgerald JF, Smith DM, Martin DK, Freedman JA, Katz BP. A case manager intervention to reduce readmissions. *Arch Intern Med* 1994; **154**: 1721–9.

36 Naylor M, Brooten D, Jones R, Lavizzo-Mourey R, Mezey M, Pauley M. Comprehensive discharge planning for the hospitalized elderly. *J Am Geriatr Soc* 1994; **120**: 999–1006.

37 Thomas DR, Brahan R, Haywood BP. Inpatient community-based geriatric assessment reduces subsequent mortality. 1993; **41**: 101–4.

38 Evans RL, Hendricks RD. Evaluating hospital discharge planning: a randomized clinical trial. *Med Care* 1993; **31**: 358–70.

39 Winograd CH, Gerety MB, Lai NA. A negative trial of impatient geriatric consultation. *Arch Intern Med* 1993; **153**: 2017–23.

40 Rubin CD, Sizemore MT, Loftis PA, Adams-Huet B, Anderson RJ. The effect of geriatric evaluation and management on medicare reimbursement in a large public hospital: a randomized clinical trial. *J Am Geriatr Soc* 1992; **40**: 989–95.

41 Hansen FR, Spedtsberg K, Schroll M. Geriatric follow-up by home visits after discharge from hospital: a randomised controlled trial. *Age Ageing* 1992; **21**: 445–50.

42 Smith DM, Weinberger M, Katz BP, Moore PS. Postdischarge care and readmissions. *Med Care* 1988; **26**: 699–708.

43 Townsend J, Piper M, Frank AO, Dyer S, North WRS, Meade TW. Reduction in hospital readmission stay of elderly patients by a community based hospital discharge scheme: a randomised controlled trial. *Br Med J* 1988; **297**: 20–7.

44 Mold JW, Stein HF. The cascade effect in clinical care of patients. *N Engl J Med* 1986; **314**: 512–14.
45 Rich MW. Heart failure disease management: a critical review. *J Card Fail* 1999; **5**: 64–75.
46 Stewart S, Pearson S, Horowitz JD. Effects of a home-based intervention among patients with chronic congestive heart failure. *Arch Intern Med* 1998; **158**: 1067–72.
47 Stewart S, Vandenbroek A, Pearson S, Horowitz J. Prolonged beneficial effects of a home-based intervention on unplanned readmissions and mortality among congestive heart failure patients. *Arch Intern Med* 1999; **159**: 257–61.
48 Kornowski R, Zeeli D, Averbuch M *et al*. Intensive home-care surveillance prevents hospitalization and improves morbidity rates among elderly patients with severe congestive heart failure. *Am Heart J* 1995; **129**: 162–6.
49 West J, Miller N, Parker K, Senneca D, et al. A comprehensive management system for heart failure improves clinical outcomes and reduces medical resource utilization. *Am J Cardiol* 1997; **79**: 58–63.
50 Fonarow GC, Stevenson LW, Walden JA *et al*. Impact of a comprehensive heart failure management program on hospital readmissions and functional status of patients with advanced heart failure. *J Am Coll Cardiol* 1997; **30**: 725–32.
51 Shah NB, Der E, Ruggerio C, Heindenreich PA, Massie BM. Prevention of hospitalizations for heart failure with an interactive home monitoring program. *Am Heart J* 1998; **135**: 373–8.

4: The increasing role of nurses in the management of heart failure in the USA

KAREN H MARTENS

In 1989 the Agency for Health Care Policy and Research was created with the goal of developing clinical guidelines to be used by health-care practitioners in the USA as an aid to effective and appropriate management of targeted clinical conditions. Heart failure, not surprisingly, was one of the first topics to be published by the Agency,[1] and these guidelines are followed in many of the programmes described in the literature. The challenges associated with managing the care of people with congestive heart failure have received considerable attention in the USA in recent years, and nurses specialised in the care of patients with cardiac problems consistently have been involved in programmes to address these issues.

This chapter represents an overview of the burden of heart failure in the USA and the development of specialist nurse-led programmes in the management of heart failure.

Background

Funding issues

With the introduction of Diagnostic Related Groups in 1983 a significant change in illness care funding was initiated which subsequently led to massive changes in the US health-care delivery. Diagnostic Related Groups changed the payment for hospital care from a retrospective payment system to a prospective one. For the first time, hospitals had limits placed on the costs of illness care, which necessitated examination of the care provided for people with diagnoses most often resulting in hospitalisation. Because chronic heart failure was and continues to be a leading reason for hospitalisation, it soon became a focus of attention; for example, patients with chronic heart failure were hospitalised for shorter periods and were increasingly referred for home healthcare services in the years between 1983 and 1986.[1,2]

Trends in heart failure hospitalisation

In 1990, the trends in hospitalisation rates for chronic heart failure within the USA during the years 1973–86 were reported to have increased annually.[3] Four groups were studied: non-white women had the largest increase in discharges (143%), followed by white women (127%), non-white men (118%), and white men (99%). Age-adjusted rates were found to be more similar for the four groups: 88% for white women, 66% for white men, 65% for non-white women, and 53% for non-white men. These increases are thought to be related to the advancing average age of the population and the increased survival rate among persons with cardiac disease. Currently, congestive (chronic) heart failure is the most prevalent admitting diagnosis in US hospitals for persons older than 65 years.[4]

The genesis of new programmes for limiting hospital use in heart failure

Discharge planning was the first line of defence used in an effort to compensate for the shortened hospital stays resulting from the introduction of the prospective payment system in 1983. Many comprehensive discharge programmes for older adults in general were developed in the late 1980s and early 1990s. Nurses or social workers continue to carry out this function in hospitals for patients at high risk of complications or readmission to the hospital, and people with chronic heart failure fall into this category.

Beginning with the early efforts of discharge planning, continual changes have taken place in the USA health-care delivery system in efforts to control costs by better management. Competition among healthcare providers appeared early in these changes, followed by mergers between hospitals and other health care agencies. Mergers continue to take place as large corporations strive to capture significant market shares of the health-care business. Health care in the United States is clearly big business. Today, discharge planning remains important in the mix of strategies used to manage the care of people with chronic heart failure, across the continuum of care; from hospital to home, where follow-up care may be provided by chronic heart failure centres, clinics, or home-care agencies. Today's managed care market is challenging health-care agencies to limit costs while at the same time maintaining or even improving the quality of care.

Delaying or preventing hospital readmission is the primary goal in the management of chronic heart failure. In the USA, people with chronic heart failure (most of whom are over 65 years old) are readmitted to hospital within 30–90 days at a rate about twice that of all elderly adults.[5] Because hospital care is the most costly of health-care services, it is desirable to limit such care as much as possible without sacrificing the health of the public. Within the climate of the changing health-care industry in the USA, it is not surprising that many strategies and programmes aimed at people with chronic heart failure have been developed with the ultimate intent of decreasing hospital usage. The annual cost of hospital care for people with chronic heart failure is about US$4 billion, and the cost of outpatient visits and medications may be equally high.[6] Because over 2 million Americans have heart failure and approximately 400 000 new cases are diagnosed each year, any reduction in hospital usage will have a significant effect on health-care costs.

Many programmes and strategies have been developed and published in an effort to improve the management of chronic heart failure. It is also true that many unpublished programs have been implemented. In reviewing the current pattern of the management of chronic heart failure in the USA through a literature review and consultation with nurses practising in this area, several trends are evident:

- Increasingly, multidisciplinary approaches are used to manage the chronic heart failure population. Nurses are essential members of multidisciplinary teams planning and delivering these comprehensive programmes. Other disciplines commonly involved include medicine, social work, health education, pharmacy, and nutrition.
- Chronic heart failure strategies frequently cross agency boundaries and span the continuum of care. This is especially true in the ever-increasing number of large, integrated delivery networks.
- Education is a key component of any comprehensive strategy directed at chronic heart failure.
- There is an increased emphasis on measuring outcomes of care.

These trends are increasingly reflected in the many chronic heart failure management approaches developed during the 1990s and discussed here.

Comprehensive heart failure programmes

Cost containment through managed care has led to the development of comprehensive heart failure programmes that include both inpatient and outpatient care strategies. Nurses play a key role in these comprehensive programmes, helping in their development as well as acting as programme coordinator, case manager, educator, and outcome evaluator. Advanced practice nurses sometimes participate in the long-term management of patients in clinics.[7] In a comprehensive programme reported by the Midwest Heart Research Foundation,[8] a clinical nurse specialist and two registered nurses formed part of a multidisciplinary team which implemented treatment protocols for both inpatients and outpatients. The team also included a cardiologist, a dietitian, a patient care technician, and a social worker. The inpatient protocol consisted of a clinical pathway with an expected length of stay of 4 days. The protocol included a broad range of strategies:

- consultations with a cardiologist, dietitian, social worker, pastoral services, and a clinical nurse specialist
- tests and treatments such as cardiac monitoring, daily weighing, strict intake and output, blood analysis, left ventricular function, and intravenous access
- medications such as angiotensin-converting enzyme (ACE) inhibitors, vasodilators, diuretics, digoxin, and intravenous inotropes
- dietary restrictions of sodium and fluids
- progressive cardiac rehabilitation
- education about signs and symptoms of chronic heart failure, medications, diet, and exercise
- discharge planning involving daily multidisciplinary rounds, home health, the outpatient chronic heart failure centre, and a support group.

Medical and nursing staff were educated about the management of chronic heart failure through the protocols. Nursing staff education emphasised important elements of the programme regimen such as the daily recording of weight, and monitoring sodium and fluid restriction. Patients and their families were taught the signs and symptoms of chronic heart failure, the importance of taking medication as prescribed, and the benefits of sodium restriction and regular exercise. A personalised medication schedule was given to each patient along with a weight-recording chart. All patients received follow-up telephone contact weekly for 1 month and then every other week for at least 90 days following hospital discharge. Patients who were at high risk of decompensation were referred to an outpatient clinic, which administered intermittent intravenous inotropes. This nurse-managed programme was highly successful, with significant decreases in length of hospital stay (22% reduction), admission rate, readmission rates (13% in the programme group), and costs to both the patient and provider.

This programme has several features in common with other comprehensive programmes that have been reported:[4, 7, 9, 10] they all use a multidisciplinary approach; case management with the aid of clinical pathways; intensive education of patients, families, and health-care professionals; and aggressive management of the clinical status of patients after hospital discharge.

The multidisciplinary approach

Several multidisciplinary efforts to manage chronic heart failure have been reported.[7-11] Teams generally include cardiologists, cardiac clinical nurse specialists, dietitians, and social workers. Services of pharmacists, rehabilitation specialists, home-care nurses, mental health counsellors, and pastoral care are sometimes also noted. Nurses participating in multidisciplinary teams may be clinical nurse specialists with postgraduate qualifications, cardiac staff nurses, discharge planners, and home-care nurses. In one programme the cardiac clinical nurse specialist provides support, education, and consultation to the heart failure team members. The expertise of the nurse is credited as being vital to the success of the programme.[4] Accordingly, nursing educators are currently being directed to prepare nurses who can function in a collaborative and interdisciplinary fashion.

Because chronic heart failure affects all aspects of the patient's life, the contributions offered through this multifaceted approach have positive outcomes in many areas. These include patient satisfaction, functional status, and cost containment as recognised in decreased length of initial hospital stay, decreased hospital readmission rate, and decreased number of hospital days. One heart failure service continues to collect longitudinal data in order to measure patient compliance with treatment regimen, symptom management, cardiac function, physical function, and quality of life.[7] Already, improvement in quality of life measured 3 months after entry into the service has been identified.

Case management

Case management, routinely used in chronic heart failure programmes, is an approach in which a nurse case manager oversees or coordinates the care of the person with chronic heart failure. Case management is concerned with cost savings and control of resource consumption, while at the same time providing good-quality patient outcomes and patient satisfaction. Case management models for chronic heart failure[12-17] these have several components in common.

Outcome measurement

A variety of outcomes are measured to determine their relationship to the use of clinical pathways. Length of hospital stay is a standard outcome measure and has been shown to decrease significantly after implementation of case management. Length of stay for patients hospitalised with chronic heart failure has been reduced significantly in several studies. Topp and colleagues compared the effects of case management performed by clinical nurse specialists in collaboration with cardiologists, with the effects of usual care.[17] The case management patients had a significantly shorter average length of stay (4.6 days v 6.29 days). Morrison and Beckworth reported a mean length of stay of 5.44 (SD 4.1) days and noted that 68% of subjects had a length of stay of 5 days or less.[16] Ball and Peruzzi reported that the average length of stay decreased from 8 days in 1994 to 5 days in 1996 as an outcome of case management.[12] Hospital readmission within 31 days also decreased from 39% in 1994 to 32% in 1996. Barrella and Della Monica reported a hospital readmission rate of only 12% within 90 days of discharge.[4] Other outcomes that have been measured after implementing case management include: functional health status, the frequency of measuring daily weight, intake, and output;[4] left ventricular ejection fraction, health knowledge, complication rates, mortality, patient satisfaction, physiological status, physical functioning, health knowledge, and family caregiver status;[16] and also costs of care.[12, 17]

Clinical pathways

Clinical pathways, also called critical pathways or care maps, are essential components of case management. A clinical pathway is a guide to the delivery of appropriate services and care in a timely manner. These pathways or maps consist of a written plan of care that is to be followed within specified time frames. Clinical pathways are expected to describe the typical course of care for 75% of patients with a specified diagnosis. They were first used in hospital settings for persons with chronic heart failure and are increasingly being used in home care.[13, 14] The literature provides numerous specific examples of pathways used in practice.[4, 10, 12, 13, 18]

Education

Education is essential if patients are to manage their chronic heart failure.[1] Because hospitalisation typically lasts between 4 to 6 days, there is insufficient time to educate patients fully about managing their chronic heart failure prior to hospital discharge. Accordingly, educational approaches are being developed that begin in the hospital and continue after discharge, following the patient through different levels of care such as home care or clinic-based programmes. Family members should be included in education and participate in the development of the plan of care.[4] Lasater reported that patient knowledge about medications is notably lacking. Also, it was found that although patients generally took their medications as prescribed, 10% used time-released glyceryl trinitrate (nitroglycerine) patches incorrectly by applying them every 4–6 hours.[10] Nurses are often the primary source of patient education in all settings, in hospitals as well as in community-based settings such as chronic heart failure clinics and home care. Although reports of chronic heart failure programmes now routinely stress the importance of patient and family education,[4, 8, 10, 13, 18–21] there is limited detail about the specific teaching methods. However, it is clear that education has had a positive impact in the management of chronic heart failure.

One patient education pathway for persons with chronic heart failure helped to halve hospital readmissions and saved the hospital $173 000.[21] Another programme, followed patients from the hospital into home-care services or long-term care settings.[18] This approach is one of care management as opposed to case management, noting that the chronic heart failure population needs continuity of care owing to the "progressive downward trajectory pattern and cyclic phasing through crises, acute, stable and unstable phases".[18] The interdisciplinary team included a publisher of health and safety materials, who helped produce a teaching packet that was mailed to physician offices, long-term care settings, home health agencies, and patients themselves when admitted to hospital, in an effort to provide continuity in what was being taught to patients and their families. Smoot has provided a comprehensive teaching handout to guide patients in managing their chronic heart failure during the first few weeks after hospital discharge.[18] It provides information and guidelines about what chronic heart failure is, when to call the doctor, when to call the emergency services, diet, exercise, smoking, drinking, medications, water retention and weight, taking a pulse measurement, and glyceryl trinitrate use.

Topics addressed through patient educational components of programmes consistently include information about:

- chronic heart failure and its associated signs and symptoms
- disease management
- medications (actions, doses, side effects, interactions, precautions, special instructions)
- low-sodium diet
- limiting alcohol and fluid intake
- the importance of balancing exercise and energy conservation
- taking and recording weight daily
- signs and symptoms to report to the nurse or doctor
- when and how to call an emergency number.

One Ohio-based home-care agency has extensive educational materials for people with chronic heart failure. Such resource materials are increasingly being used by home-care agencies. This agency provided:

- pamphlets about a "no added salt" diet, potassium, and seasoning food without salt
- a patient care calendar that provides information about the goals of nursing care, teaching points, and when the chronic heart failure will be considered stable

- multiple handouts about a variety of topics related to managing chronic heart failure.

Educational interventions are delivered in a variety of ways. Educational materials are frequently designed especially for the chronic heart failure population and even personalised for individual patients. One programme sends patients four educational packets to their homes after discharge, each with a personalised cover letter; these packets use a variety of formats to catch the attention of the patients. Another strategy uses teaching videotapes. Teaching checklists sometimes are used to enable caregivers to know what points have been taught to hospitalised patients, to ensure that all essential topics have been covered during the hospital stay. Personalised medication schedules are sometimes developed to help patients comply with prescribed medication regimens. Medication containers are provided cheaply or free to help people organise their medications according to the time of day they are to be taken. One programme gives patients a satchel to carry their medications in when they return to the heart centre for follow-up care. Because daily weighing is crucial in managing chronic heart failure, it is important to determine if a patient owns a scale, and some programmes will give patients a scale if they do not. Also, charts are provided for recording and tracking daily weights.

Clinical management

Clinical management is the monitoring of symptoms and the provision of treatment to prevent problems as well as to treat them. With chronic heart failure patients, the goal is to identify problems early so as to prevent suffering, rehospitalisation, and possibly death. The most successful chronic heart failure programmes use an aggressive approach through frequent follow-up of patients. Whilst physicians determine medical treatment, it is necessary that nurses and physicians work collaboratively in order to prevent acute cardiac decompensation. The nurses' role in clinical management may include a variety of functions such as monitoring clinical status, providing education, and implementing medical treatments. While it is not the intent here to provide details of clinical management, some general information may be of interest.

Patients in the multidisciplinary programmes are monitored closely. Efforts are made to establish rapid contact with patients following discharge from hospital. Patients may be monitored by nurses in home visits, clinic care, telephone follow-up, or a combination of strategies. For instance, patients may be seen weekly after discharge until they are medically stable; visits to see a physician can then become less frequent. Patients with advanced chronic heart failure (New York Heart Association class III or IV) may receive outpatient intravenous inotrope infusions.

Home care is a frequently used strategy for monitoring the clinical status of patients with chronic heart failure and has been associated with a lower hospital readmission rate.[22] Home-care agencies are increasingly developing disease management programmes for patients with common diagnoses.

One highly successful programme was developed by a cardiac clinical nurse specialist and staffed by nurses experienced in critical care.[4] The programme follows a clinical pathway based on Agency for Health Care Policy and Research recommendations. Of 92 patients, only 11 (12%) were readmitted to the hospital within 90 days. The programme includes comprehensive cardiopulmonary assessment, extensive patient education, intravenous diuretic administration, inotropic therapy, laboratory services, electrocardiograph monitoring, and pulse oximetry when indicated. This clinic also uses a few strategies not routinely reported. A psychiatric clinical nurse specialist is available to provide supportive counselling to non-compliant and depressed patients. Also, the heart failure team meets weekly to discuss issues and strategies for patients with more complex problems. They believe that the care of the chronic heart failure patient requires a team approach, with the patient at the centre; nevertheless, the cardiac clinical nurse specialist is also seen as vital to the programme's success.

Singh offers an assessment and intervention checklist for home-care nurses managing the care of patients with chronic heart failure.[23] This thorough checklist is presented in conjunction with a case study that effectively illustrates the potential need for these actions (see box).

Assessment checklist for management of patients with chronic heart failure at home:

- cardiac history
- level of consciousness
- blood pressure
- pulse characteristics
- neck vein distension
- bruits
- chest auscultation for adventitious sounds
- cough, shortness of breath on exertion
- orthopnoea
- oedema
- skin characteristics
- cyanosis, pale
- weakness, dizziness, tiredness
- low urine output
- liver enlargement
- ascites

(From Singh[23])

Intervention possibilities were identified as:

- making breathing easier
- promoting rest
- elevating feet
- raising patient from a lying to a standing position
- providing emotional support
- monitoring weight
- instructing on skin care
- providing nutritional education
- monitoring elimination
- instructing on and monitoring medications.

Clinic care is also used to monitor clinical status. One nurse-managed chronic heart failure clinic, developed in collaboration with attending cardiologists, has also been successful in significantly reducing hospital readmission rates and the length of hospital stay.[10] The clinic operates on a chronic complex illness model of care, which recognises that there are multiple contributing factors to disease, and the aim of intervention is improvement. The patient is an active participant in a continuous process of care. All patients discharged from the hospital with chronic heart failure are automatically admitted to the nursing clinic. The clinic protocol includes approaches congruent with other strategies discussed in this chapter:

- a complete cardiopulmonary assessment
- daily weighing
- patient education about medication and a sodium-restricted diet
- assessment of medication compliance
- assistance with financial constraints.

Conclusion

Since the 1980s, management of chronic heart failure in the USA has changed dramatically. Whilst there is still room for improvement in the management of chronic heart failure for many individuals, considerable advances have been made. Numerous approaches have been implemented in an effort to maintain optimal functional status and prevent chronic heart failure progression, which has so often resulted in cyclic admissions to the hospital. Nurses have been consistently involved in designing strategies to improve the management of people with chronic heart failure. Implemented strategies are increasingly comprehensive and provided across the continuum of care. Most recently, "disease management" has been seen as an emerging trend in managing the care of common health problems, including chronic heart failure.

Disease management is a coordinated, proactive, disease-specific approach to patient care that seeks to produce the best clinical outcomes in the most cost-effective manner. Disease management programmes also span the continuum of care, including hospital-based care, home-based care, and long-term institutional care. This is especially true in the ever-increasing number of large integrated delivery networks. Such networks include a variety of health-care settings such as hospitals, nursing homes, home-care agencies, clinics, hospices, pharmacies, medical equipment supply companies, and rehabilitation settings.

The goal of disease management is to decrease health-care costs by eliminating unnecessary hospital use while at the same time improving the quality of life.[4] Disease management incorporates a case management approach but also relies on data analysis, practice guidelines, provider and patient education, and outcomes assessment.[19] Thus, such programmes focus on improving measurable outcomes of care such as the percentage of patients who have documented daily weights, improved functional health status, patient satisfaction, and hospital use. Laing and Behrendt reported a disease management programme for home-care patients with chronic heart failure that involved home-care visits and follow-up telephone calls over the period of 1 year.[19] It is clear that nurses have played an essential role in the management of patients with chronic heart failure for many years. Now they have also become major partners in developing programmes of care and related analysis of outcomes through research. Indeed, the success of one such programme has been attributed to extensive research, development, and planning.[4]

It would be misleading to imply that all, or even most, of the people in the USA who have heart failure have their care managed through multidisciplinary programmes as described here. Unfortunately, there is still much to be done. However, the development and subsequent success of the many efforts by nurses and other health-care professionals have demonstrated effective disease management strategies. Programmes such as those described here hold much promise for improving the quality of life for the hundreds of thousands of persons living with chronic heart failure in the USA.

References

1   Agency for Health Care Policy and Research. *Heart failure: evaluation and care of patients with left-ventricular systolic dysfunction.* US Department of Health and Human Services, 1994.
2   Rich MW, Freedland, KE. Effect of DRGs on three-month readmission rate of geriatric patients with congestive heart failure. *Am J Publ Health* 1988; **78**: 680–2.
3   Ghali JK, Cooper R, Ford E. Trends in hospitalization rates for heart failure in the United States, 1973–1986. *Arch Intern Med* 1990; **150**: 769–73.
4   Barrella P, Della Monica E. Managing congestive heart failure at home. *AACN Clin Iss* 1998; **9**: 377–88.
5   Vinson JM, Rich MW, Sperry JC, Shah AS, McNamara T. Early readmission of elderly

patients with congestive heart failure. *J Am Geriatr Soc* 1990; **38**: 1290–5.

6 Funk M, Krumholz HM. Epidemiologic and economic impact of advanced heart failure. *J Cardiovasc Nurs* 1996; **10**: 1–10.

7 Urden LD. Heart failure collaborative care: an integrated partnership to manage quality and outcomes. *Outcomes Man Nurs Pract* 1998; **2**: 64–70.

8 Rauh RA, Schwabauer NJ, Enger EL, Moran JF. A community hospital-based congestive heart failure program: impact on length of stay, admission and readmission rates, and cost. *Am J Man Care* 1999; **5**: 37–43.

9 Chapman DB, Torpy J. Development of a heart failure center: a medical center and cardiology practice join forces to improve care and reduce costs. *Am J Man Care* 1997; **3**: 431–7.

10 Lasater M. The effect of a nurse-managed CHF clinic on patient readmission and length of stay. *Home Health Nurse* 1996; **5**: 351–6.

11 Venner GH, Seelbinder JS. Team management of congestive heart failure across the continuum. *J Cardiovasc Nurs* 1996; **10**: 71–84.

12 Ball C, Peruzzi M. Case management improves congestive heart failure outcomes. *Nurs Case Man* 1997; **2**: 68–74.

13 Goodwin DR. Critical pathways in home healthcare. *J Nurs Adm* 1992; **22**: 35–40.

14 Huggins CM, Phillips CY. Using case management with clinical plans to improve patient outcomes. *Home Health Nurse* 1998; **16**: 15–20.

15 Mass S, Johnson B. Case management and clinical guidelines. *J Care Man* 1998; (special edn): 18–26.

16 Morrison RS, Beckworth V. Outcomes for patients with congestive heart failure in a nursing case management model. *Nurs Case Man* 1998; **3**: 108–14.

17 Topp R, Tucker D, Weber C. Effect of a clinical case manager/clinical nurse specialist on patients hospitalized with congestive heart failure. *Nurs Case Man* 1998; **3**: 140–7.

18 Smoot SM. Continuity of care prism process applied to the congestive heart failure population. *Nurs Case Man* 1998; **3**: 79–88.

19 Laing G, Behrendt D. A disease management program for home health care patients with congestive heart failure. *Home Health Care Man Pract* 1998; **10**: 27–32.

20 Hospital focus: CHF patient education across the continuum. *RN* 1999; **62**: 30D.

21 Acute care decisions: patient education. CHF education saved this hospital $173,000. *RN* 1998; **61**: 24C–D.

22 Martens KH, Mellor SD. A study of the relationship between home care services and hospital readmission of patients with congestive heart failure. *Home Health Nurse* 1997; **15**: 123–9.

23 Singh P. Managing chronic congestive heart failure in the home. *Home Health Nurse* 1995; **13**: 11–13.

5: Integrated care for patients with chronic heart failure: the New Zealand experience

ROBERT N DOUGHTY, SUE P WRIGHT, HELEN J WALSH, STEPHANIE MUNCASTER, ANN PEARL, NORMAN SHARPE

Introduction

Chronic heart failure is a major public health problem, characterised by impaired quality of life, frequent hospital admissions and poor survival. In New Zealand, a population of approximately 3.5 million, there are about 12 000 hospital admissions for heart failure each year.[1] These admissions alone account for about 1.5% of the total New Zealand health budget.[2] During the past 20 years there have been significant advances in heart failure management related to improved understanding of pathophysiology, better methods of assessment and improved drug treatments. The angiotensin converting enzyme inhibitors[3] and beta-blockers,[4, 5] for example, can provide definite symptomatic benefit and improved survival and these agents should now be part of routine treatment. However, despite compelling clinical trial evidence, they may only be used in a minority of eligible patients with heart failure.[6] There are numerous barriers recognised between presentation of clinical trial evidence and translation into practice, some of which may be removed through the use of best practice guidelines. However, the effectiveness of printed guidelines has been debated[7] and heart failure in particular, lacking convenient surrogate measures, is a complex condition and difficult to manage optimally. For any guideline to be effective, the process and aims require careful consideration and optimal management must first be clearly defined.

An important question to be addressed is "Who should best manage heart failure and where?". Encouragement of the "gatekeeper" function of primary care doctors, to minimise patient exposure to specialists and contain costs, runs counter to the trend of establishing subspecialty care centres for specific conditions such as heart failure.[8] An integrated, participatory approach involving primary and secondary care, patient and family or support persons, appears most appropriate. An appropriate comparison can be made with existent models such as those for diabetes care, asthma treatment and cancer management. The full potential benefit of modern heart failure management has yet to be provided for most patients. During the next few years, much greater improvement for patients might be achieved through better application of current treatments that are of proven benefit rather than the introduction of additional new treatments. Consistent with the aims of improving patients' symptoms, maintaining comfort and mobility, and improving survival is the potential to reduce the considerable healthcare expenditure on heart failure through reduction of hospital admissions.

Several studies have now shown that multidisciplinary, home-based interventions for patients with heart failure[9-11] can reduce hospital readmissions and improve quality of life. Education, counselling and ongoing support for patients with heart failure appear essential for effective long-term management.[12] An alternative, or perhaps complementary, approach for management of patients with heart failure is a hospital-based clinic. Specialist heart failure clinics have been advocated to improve long term management.[13] However, such clinics are expensive to run and at present are often limited to tertiary institutions with specific purposes, such as heart transplantation or research.

Management of patients with heart failure may be improved by the combined follow-up between specialists and general practitioners. Evidence of the benefits and cost-effectiveness of such management programmes is required from randomised, controlled trials including a wide range of patients before general recommendations are made. The Auckland Heart Failure Management Study was designed to determine the effects of an integrated heart failure management programme on hospital readmissions and quality of life in patients with heart failure. The preliminary results from this study, recently presented in abstract form, demonstrate an improvement in quality of life and a reduction in multiple readmissions.[14] The following sections provide a summary of the design of the study and detail of the integrated management approach that was adopted for the study.

Auckland heart failure management study

Study setting and aims

While the overall structure of the New Zealand healthcare system is similar to that of the National Health Service in the UK, primary health care differs as it is funded by a combination of patient fee-for-service and a government funded per-patient subsidy. Most patients with chronic heart failure in New Zealand are cared for primarily by their general practitioner. Thus we considered that integration of primary and secondary care might be an effective management strategy in our healthcare setting. The aim of this study was to assess in a randomised controlled trial, the benefits of a comprehensive approach to heart failure management. Specifically, an integrated and participatory management approach involving primary and secondary care, patient and family and incorporating clinical review, standardised treatment, education, counselling and planned follow-up.

Study design

Patients considered for this trial were those admitted to Auckland Hospital with a principal diagnosis of heart failure. Exclusion criteria were kept to a minimum to allow a wide range of patients to be enrolled:

- a surgically remediable cause for heart failure (such as severe aortic stenosis)
- consideration for heart transplantation
- inability to provide informed consent
- terminal cancer
- participation in any other clinical trial.

Potentially eligible patients were reviewed and recruited into the study during their hospital stay. Patients were randomised to either the intervention group (see below) or control group. Contamination of the control group management may have occurred if a general practitioner had patients in both groups. Thus cluster randomisation was performed with the general practitioner as the unit of randomisation. In this way, each general practitioner had patients assigned to only one or other group in the study.

Although patients were identified during an in-patient stay, the study team had no input into the medical management of the patients prior to discharge. Thus the study commenced from the time of discharge following the index admission, although the actual intervention (see below) was delayed until the first outpatient visit following discharge.

Patients were randomised to either the intervention group ($n = 100$) or the control group ($n = 97$), with follow up for 12 months (Figure 5.1). The intervention group involved integrated of care between the patient/family, a hospital-based heart failure clinic and the general practitioner. This management programme is discussed further below. Patients randomised to the control group continued under the care of their general practitioner with additional follow-up measures as recommended by the medical team responsible for their in-patient care.

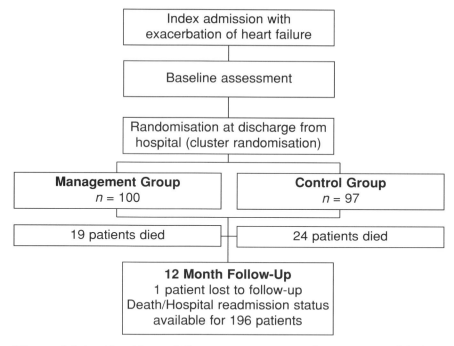

Figure 5.1 Auckland heart failure management study: summary of design.

Primary end-points for the study were:

a) combined end-point of death or hospital readmission (time to first event) and
b) quality of life (Minnesota Living with Heart Failure questionnaire.[15]

Secondary end-points included:

a) all-cause hospital readmissions
b) total hospital bed days and
c) readmissions for worsening heart failure.

The management programme (Intervention Group)

The patients in the intervention group were cared for in a shared-care arrangement between the hospital-based clinic and the patient's own general practitioner. The patient's GP was contacted at the time of randomisation by letter and by telephone to discuss the study and the plans for follow-up. A clinical review at the hospital clinic was arranged for within 2 weeks of discharge. A standard approach was taken at each clinic visit (see below).

Clinical status review

At the initial clinic review all available clinical information from the hospital admission was reviewed and possible remediable and exacerbating factors checked. Regular clinical reviews included assessment of symptoms and signs of heart failure, body weight, and repeat blood biochemistry as required.

A cardiologist and a heart failure nurse practitioner ran this clinic. One hour was allocated for the first clinic visit, and 30–45 minutes for follow-up visits.

The clinics were held at Auckland Hospital and the most common reasons for non-attendance at the clinic were transport problems or personal reasons. The nurse practitioner at the hospital heart failure clinic was available for consultation during normal working hours and received an average of 6 calls per patient (range 0–20) during the 12 month follow-up.

Pharmacological treatment

A standardised approach to combination treatment with diuretic agents, angiotensin converting enzyme inhibitors and digoxin was applied with individualisation as appropriate according to clinical review and investigative findings. Contemporary clinical practice guidelines were used to provide a standard approach to pharmacological treatment.[16] The study recruited patients during 1997–8, prior to the publication of the definitive ß-blocker trials, and thus the frequency of ß-blockers use was low. The patient kept a medication record with any changes noted and a weekly record of all medication taken to allow monitoring of compliance.

Patient education and counselling

A specialist nurse-practitioner initiated education and counselling of the patient and family at the first clinic visit on an individual basis. The aims were to assist patient understanding of the symptoms and signs of heart failure, body weight monitoring, indications of worsening heart failure, effects of medications and recommendations on diet and activity. An explanatory heart failure booklet was provided, along with the patient diary containing weight and medication records (see below).

Three group education sessions were offered for the intervention group, two within 6 weeks of entry into the study and the third after 6 months. Seventy percent of the intervention group attended the first group education session, and 47% attended the 6 month session. Each session lasted for about one and a half hours and was run predominately by the nurse practitioner. Family members or other support persons were invited to attend and active participation during the sessions was encouraged. The content of the one-on-one and group education included:

- explanation of the symptoms and signs of heart failure
- importance of monitoring of daily body weight and action plans should weight change
- effects of medications and importance of compliance
- recommendations regarding exercise, diet, smoking and alcohol.

The advice given was individualised and reinforced at each subsequent clinic visit or group session. The sessions were informal and attendance kept to 8 to 12 people so that recommendations could be individualised.

Patient diary

Patients were given a personal diary in which there was space to record contact details, appointment times, medication record and a week by week diary to record daily weight and any change in symptoms. A heart failure information booklet (New Zealand Heart Foundation) was also given to each patient and provided written information regarding symptoms, medications, weight, diet, exercise, and other practical information. The diary became an essential part of the patient's self-management programme.

Follow up plan

A clearly defined individualised follow-up plan was discussed and defined with the patient and family/support at the first clinic visit. The recommendations were for patients to have six weekly checks alternating with the GP and hospital clinic. After all clinic visits a summary letter was faxed to the GP on the same day and specific notes made of any recommended changes. Patients were instructed to contact their GP in the first instance in the case of worsening symptoms. The GP was free to manage each patient as they saw appropriate but discussion regarding management difficulties was encouraged. A member of the heart failure team was easily contactable by the GP during normal working hours. GPs were able to fax the clinic directly and were encouraged to comment in the patient's diary at each visit. The heart failure team provided an efficient service for the GPs and an up-to-date knowledge base in heart failure management.

Place of integrated management programmes in the context of current management

The aims of this trial were to assess the effects of an integrated, participatory approach to the management of patients with chronic heart failure. The benefits of specialist heart failure clinics have been advocated,[13] although evidence is required from randomised controlled trials before such interventions are implemented. This study aimed to include the general practitioner in the management programme, as in many countries patients with heart failure are managed mainly in primary care. Optimal integration between primary and secondary care may not have been achieved in this study, although there may have been benefits not quantified by frequency of visits alone. Final publication of the full results from this trial are awaited before final recommendations can be made.

Given the importance of primary care in the management of chronic diseases in many countries, an alternative model is to facilitate increased access to primary care alone. However, a recent randomised controlled trial involving US Veterans[17] showed that this approach did not decrease hospital admissions. In this study, 1396 US Veterans with diabetes, congestive heart failure ($n = 504$) or chronic obstructive pulmonary disease were randomly assigned to either an intensive primary care intervention or usual care. The intervention involved close follow-up by a nurse and a primary care physician beginning before discharge and continuing for 6 months. The patients in the intervention group had significantly higher rates of readmission than the controls (0.19 vs. 0.14 per month respectively, p = 0.005). In addition, more patients in the intervention group had multiple readmissions than in the control group. One reason for the increase in admissions may have been the detection of previously unrecognised medical conditions that required admission for treatment. In addition, a disease specific protocol and integration of primary with specialist care, as in the Auckland study, may be important requirements for the success of such management programmes.

While the intervention trials have utilised different designs, the heart failure nurse practitioner is common to all the trials and appears to have a key role in heart failure management, whether in home-based interventions,[9–11] nurse-led hospital clinics[18] or more integrated care programmes. These nurse practitioners need to be trained in heart failure management and have access to other resources, particularly a multidisciplinary team, which may include doctors, pharmacists, and social workers.

Alternative strategies to integrate primary and secondary care may be employed. However, the strategy undertaken should be applicable to the local health care environment and be appropriately supported and resourced. It is important to remember that, whatever strategies are provided, every patient has different and distinct educational and medical needs and thus flexible and practical approaches should be employed to accommodate individual needs. Since the Auckland Study began further evidence has emerged with regard to the beneficial effects of ß-bockers[4, 5] and spironolactone.[19] These treatments need to be incorporated in integration strategies and may themselves force a change in the provision of care for patients with heart failure. For example, ß-blocker therapy while providing clear long-term benefits may also cause adverse effects. The safe use of these agents requires careful patient selection, appropriate initiation, and titration with clinical monitoring, which may not be easily facilitated in primary care. Thus, future integration strategies should carefully consider the effects of implementing these treatments.

Conclusions

Hospital admissions for heart failure have consistently increased over the last 10–20 years and the cost of these admissions alone account for 1–1.5% of total health budgets in most developed countries.[2, 20] There is thus an urgent need for strategies to reduce these admissions. Several randomised, controlled trials have now assessed different approaches in the management of patients with heart failure.[9, 10, 17, 21–23] The current study supports the role of integrated management involving the patient/family and primary and secondary care, although full details of the effects of this intervention are yet to be published. There may be benefits in combining different approaches, such as providing facilities for home-based interventions, perhaps targeting higher risk individuals whilst also providing community based education strategies and integrated primary-secondary care. However, this does extend beyond the current evidence-base and different combinations of interventions require further study. Benefits may be achieved with earlier intervention in hospital prior to discharge, use of agents proven to reduce admissions, such as ß-blocker therapy,[4, 5] and further attention to the comorbidities commonly found in these patients.

Implementation of these evidence based management programmes has the potential to improve the quality of life for patients with heart failure and reduce the public health burden of this disease. However, it should be noted that such management programmes have only been applied to patients who have been admitted to hospital. Consequently, there is no evidence of benefit in reducing the first admission for patients with newly diagnosed heart failure. In addition, the programmes have generally only followed patients for a relatively short period and the longer-term effects remain uncertain.

References

1 Doughty RN, Wright SP, Gamble G, Sharpe N. Increasing hospital admissions and decreasing length of hospital stay for heart failure in New Zealand (1988–1997). *J Cardiac Failure* 1999, 5 (Suppl 1): 63.

2 Doughty R, Yee T, Sharpe N, MacMahon S. Hospital admissions and deaths due to congestive heart failure in New Zealand, 1988-91. *NZ Med J* 1995; **108**: 473–5.

3 Garg R, Yusuf S, for the Collaborative Group on ACE Inhibitor Trials. Overview of randomised trials of angiotensin-converting enzyme inhibitors on mortality and morbidity in patients with heart failure. *JAMA* 1995; **273**: 1450–6.

4 CIBIS-II Investigators and Committees. The Cardiac Insufficiency Bisoprolol Study II

(CIBIS-II): a randomised trial. *Lancet* 1999; **353**: 9–13.

5   MERIT-HF Study Group. Effect of metoprolol CR/XL in chronic heart failure: metoprolol CR/XL randomised intervention trial in congestive heart failure (MERIT-HF). *Lancet* 1999; **353**: 2001–7.

6   Rajfer SI. Perspective of the pharmaceutical industry on the development of new drugs for heart failure. *J Am Coll Cardiol* 1993; **22** (Suppl A): 198A–200A.

7   Tunis SR, Hayward RSA, Wilson MC, Rubin HR, Bass EB, Johnson M, *et al.* Internists attitudes about clinical practice guidelines. *Ann Intern Med* 1994; **120**: 956–3.

8   Kronick R, Goodman DC, Weenberg J, Wagner E. The market place for health reform. *N Eng J Med* 1993; **328**: 148–52.

9   Rich MWR, Beckham V, Wittenberg C, Leyen CL, Freedland KE, Carney RM. A multidisciplinary intervention to prevent the readmission of elderly patients with congestive heart failure. *N Engl J Med* 1995; **333**: 1190–5.

10 Stewart S, Pearson S, Horowitz JD. Effects of a home-based intervention among patients with congestive heart failure discharged from acute hospital care. *Arch Int Med* 1998; **158**: 1067–72.

11 Stewart S, Marley JE, Horowiz JD. Effects of a multidisciplinary, homebased intervention on unplanned readmissions and survival among patients with chronic congestive heart failure: a randomised, controlled study. *Lancet* 1999; **354**: 1077–83.

12 Jaarsma T, Halfens R, Abu-Saad HH, Dracup K, Gorgels T, van Ree J, *et al.* Effects of education and support on self-care and resource utilisation in patients with heart failure. *Eur Heart J* 1999; **20**: 673–82.

13 Abraham WT, Bristow MR. Specialised centers for heart failure management. *Circulation* 1997; **96**: 2755–7.

14 Doughty RN, Wright S, Walsh H, Muncaster S, Whalley G, Gamble G, *et al.* The Auckland Heart Failure Management Study: a randomised controlled trial of integrated heart failure management (abstract). *J Cardiac Failure* 1999; **5** (Suppl 1): 50.

15 Rector TS, Kubo SH, Cohn JN. Patients self-assessment of their congestive heart failure: content, reliability and validity of a new measure – the Minnesota Living with Heart Failure questionnaire. *Heart Failure* 1987; **3**: 198–209.

16 Agency for Health Care Policy and Research. *Heart failure: evaluation and care of patients with left-ventricular systolic dysfunction.* US Department of Health and Human Services, 1994.

17 Weinberger M, Oddone EZ, Henderson WG, for the Veterans Affairs Cooperative Study Group on Primary Care and Hospital Readmission. Does increased access to primary care reduce hospital readmissions? *N Eng J Med* 1996; **334**: 1441–7.

18 Cline CMJ, Israelsson BYA, Willenheimer RB, Broms K, Erhardt LR. Cost effective management programme for heart failure reduces hospitalisation. *Heart* 1998; **80**: 442–6.

19 Pitt B, Zannad F, Remme WJ, Cody R, Castaigne A, Perez A, *et al.* The effects of spironolactone on morbidity and mortality in patients with severe heart failure. Randomized Aldactone Evaluation Study Investigators. *N Engl J Med* 1999; **341**: 709–17.

20 McMurray J, Hart W, Rhodes G. An evaluation of the cost of heart failure to the National Health Service in the UK. *Br J Med Econ* 1993; **6**: 99–110.

21 Schneider JK, Hornberger S, Booker J, Davis A, Kralicek R. A medication discharge planning programme: measuring the effect on readmissions. *Clin Nurs Res* 1993; **2**: 41–53.

22 Serxner S, Miyaji M, Jeffords J. Congestive heart failure disease management study: a patient education intervention. *Congestive Heart Fail* 1998; **4**: 23–8.

23 Gattis WA, Hasselblad V, Whellan DJ, O'Connor CM. Reduction in heart failure events by the addition of a clinical pharmacist intervention to the heart failure management team. Results of the Pharmacist in Heart Failure Assessment Recommendation and Monitoring (PHARM) Study. *Arch Intern Med* 1999; **159**: 1939–45.

Acknowledgements

The study was funded by a project grant from the National Heart Foundation of New Zealand and an unrestricted educational grant from Merck Sharp Dohme (NZ) Ltd. RND is the recipient of the New Zealand National Heart Foundation BNZ Senior Fellowship.

6: Nurse-led clinics for the management of heart failure in Sweden

CHARLES CLINE, ANNELI IWARSON

In Sweden, as in other developed countries, heart failure represents a major health-care concern with regard to incidence, prevalence, mortality, morbidity, and health-care costs. Conservative estimates suggest that there are more than 100 000 patients suffering from heart failure due to left ventricular systolic dysfunction and that the number with asymptomatic systolic left ventricular dysfunction is three to four times as great. In addition, heart failure with preserved systolic left ventricular function is common, especially in elderly people and women. This condition cannot be clinically differentiated from heart failure due to systolic dysfunction and is estimated to account for about 30% of all cases of heart failure. Thus, the incidence of heart failure in Sweden is in excess of 160 000, which constitutes 2% of the population.

Heart failure results in severe impairment of quality of life comparable to the most debilitating chronic diseases, and is associated with a frequent need for hospitalisation. Hospitalisation is the major single cause of the health-care costs associated with heart failure. Also, despite advances in the treatment of heart failure, it remains in many cases a serious disease carrying a poor prognosis. Given the system for health care in Sweden, there has been growing interest in improving the management of heart failure in order to improve prognosis, reduce morbidity, improve quality of life, and – importantly, in a situation with insufficient health-care resources – reduce expenditure. The aim of this chapter is to describe, against the background of the Swedish health-care system, the development of management strategies for heart failure in Sweden from research to implementation in present-day clinical practice.

The health-care system in Sweden

In Europe there are, in principle, two systems for financing health care. On the one hand there is an insurance-based system such as in Germany, the Netherlands, and Belgium. On the other hand there is a tax-based system, which is the system used in the UK, Sweden, and the other Scandinavian countries. All people residing in Sweden are covered to a similar extent by a national, tax-financed health-care insurance. The benefits of this insurance are independent of the amount of tax each individual has (or has not) paid. In recent years Sweden has had to implement cost reductions in the health-care sector in order to ensure balance in the country's economy and also in order to be able to meet the European Union's requirements for joining the European Monetary Union. However, these cuts in expenditure have stimulated innovations aimed at more cost-effective care. In the management of heart failure, new concepts have been developed aimed not only at improving care but also at providing cost-effective management. In Sweden data from 1996 showed that the mean length of stay for heart failure in wards for internal medicine varied from 3.5 days to 9.5 days, depending on the hospital. The national average length of stay was 6.5 days. This may reflect differences in the organisation of the care for heart failure patients.

A comparison between 1990 and 1997 shows that the cost of drugs within the national health-care system has increased in Sweden from 8.4% to 14.9% of the total health-care budget. This equals an absolute increase in monetary terms of 81%. In the treatment of heart failure, however, there has been – and still is – an underprescription of recommended treatment. The use of angiotensin-converting enzyme (ACE) inhibitors and ß-blockers is cost-effective in the treatment of heart failure (at least that due to systolic left ventricular dysfunction). Indeed, in heart failure the cost of drugs amounts to only a minor part of the total cost for managing heart failure patients. Therefore, there is no reason to try to curtail an increased use of appropriate drugs in these patients.

Health-care costs for heart failure in Sweden

The total health-care cost for the management of heart failure in Sweden has been calculated to be approximately SEK2 500 million, about 2% of the total national health-care budget. The major expense in the management of heart failure is institutional care, i.e. hospitalisation and nursing home care (Figure 6.1). Heart failure is in fact the fourth most common reason for hospital care and the most common reason in patients over the age of 65 years in Sweden. Furthermore, heart failure accounts for 14% of all hospitalisations for diseases of the circulatory system.[1]

The mean length of stay in hospital for heart failure varies within Sweden. It may initially seem that hospitals with short durations of stay are more effective. However, in some circumstances at least, short stays are associated

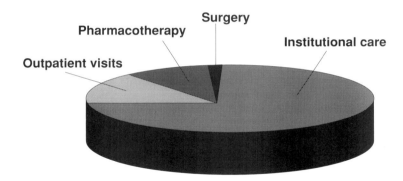

igure 6.1 The relative expenditure on direct costs for heart failure management (adapted from Bergsten-Ryden T *et al.*[1]).

with a higher risk of readmission.[2] In one study patients readmitted within 30 days were found to have a significantly shorter median length of stay than patients not readmitted within 1 year. It has been suggested that this may be due to inadequate time spent in stabilising patients or preparing for adequate follow-up after discharge. These are important factors that have been addressed in a number of studies of heart failure management in an attempt to improve care and reduce the rates of readmission.

Outpatient care accounts for only a small proportion of the total cost of managing heart failure patients, in fact only 6%.[1] It has been estimated that on average heart failure patients make three or four outpatient visits to their primary care physician annually. Heart failure is one of the ten most common reasons for visits to primary care physicians, but constitutes only 1.1% of the total number of visits; in comparison, hypertension is the most common reason and accounts for 4.4% of visits.[3]

The cost of pharmacological treatment represents approximately 11% (SEK294 million) of the total cost for heart failure.[1] The most common treatment was with diuretic drugs which were used in 78% of heart failure patients (SEK108 million), whereas the most costly treatment (SEK150 million) was the prescription of ACE inhibitors, used in only 24% of patients.

Quality of life in heart failure

Quality of life is an important aspect of heart failure management. Of course, it is important in all illnesses, since improving quality of life is one of the major aims of treatment if it is impaired. In heart failure quality of life is severely affected. Heart failure is also a disease that carries a poor prognosis. In combination with the fact that an increasing number of patients are elderly or very elderly, the ability to influence mortality rates diminishes and the importance of quality of life increases.

Quality of life is impaired in all aspects traditionally measured, for example, emotions, sleep, energy, pain, and mobility.[4] Also, the patient's social life, family life, and sex life are negatively influenced. As could be expected, quality of life deteriorates with increased disease severity. It seems to be impaired to a greater extent in women than in men, which is an unexpected finding, although similar findings have been made in other cardiac disorders.[5] The degree of impairment is comparable to other illnesses such as severe rheumatoid arthritis.

Compliance and patient education in heart failure

In Sweden as in other countries compliance is poor in heart failure patients and this often is a precipitating cause of hospitalisation. Patient compliance with drug therapy is poor, and when studied 30 days after discharge from hospital at least 25% of elderly heart failure patients were found not to comply with prescribed medication.[6]

Improving compliance has become an important part of nurse management in heart failure. Video and multimedia interactive programmes have been developed for patient education aimed at enhancing compliance among other things. In Sweden, this approach has been shown to be effective in increasing patients' knowledge about heart failure and its treatment, and it may be an effective instrument to be used by heart failure nurses.[7]

Studies of nurse-led outpatient clinics

Nurses in Sweden have a high standard of training and in many areas a tradition of working independently. In the past this may have been due to a shortage of physicians, resulting in nurses performing tasks that in other countries would ordinarily be performed by doctors. More recently it may also have been due to the lower costs involved in employing nurses rather than doctors. However, at present nurses in Sweden often have defined and specialised roles in disease management. In cardiology nurses have a well-established role in secondary prevention and therefore it is quite natural for them to take an active part in the management of heart failure. Indeed, heart failure management has developed and become as complex and as specialised as the management of acute coronary syndromes and secondary prevention.

The first randomised trial started in Sweden to evaluate the impact of a nurse-led, easy-access, heart failure outpatient clinic included 190 patients.[8,9] Patients aged 65–84 years were eligible for randomisation if they had been admitted primarily because of heart failure. The patients were randomised either to a control group followed up in accordance with clinical routine at the time, or to an intervention group followed up at a nurse-led clinic. Patients randomised to the intervention group were visited twice by a heart failure nurse during their hospital stay. The purpose of these visits was to educate patients about heart failure and heart failure treatment including flexible, patient-guided diuretic therapy based on signs and symptoms of heart failure. The patients also received a "heart failure diary" in which they could record their weight, signs and symptoms of heart failure, list of medications, instructions for increasing and decreasing diuretic dosage, as well as relevant names and telephone numbers for the heart failure clinic. Two weeks after discharge patients were invited along with their spouse, a family member or a friend to participate in a group education session led by the heart failure nurse. The previously given information was reinforced using an oral presentation, an educational video, and a question-and-answer session. During the year following discharge all intervention group patients had a minimum of two doctor's visits at 1 month and 4 months, and one nurse visit at 8 months. Patients were able to contact the study nurse at any time during office hours and, if needed, were scheduled for additional visits either to a nurse or physician depending on what was deemed appropriate.

The short-term and long-term effects of the intervention were studied according to specified end-points. In the short-term evaluation at 90 days there was a trend towards increased event-free survival in the intervention group and there was also a significant reduction in mortality (Figure 6.2). Quality of life improved significantly more in the intervention group (Figure 6.3). In the long-term follow-up at 1 year no significant differences were found with regard to survival or quality of life. However, time to readmission was increased in the intervention group (141 ± 87 days v 106 ± 100 days, p < 0.05) and hospitalisation as well as health-care costs were reduced (days hospitalised, 4.2 ± 7.8 v 8.2 ± 14.3, p = 0.07; costs, US$2 294 v US$3 594, p = 0.07).

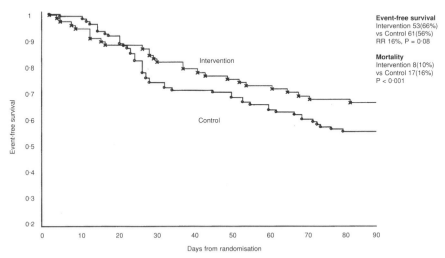

Figure 6.2 Reduction in mortality and increase in event-free survival in heart failure patients followed up at a nurse-led, outpatient clinic (intervention) compared to patients with conventional follow-up (control).

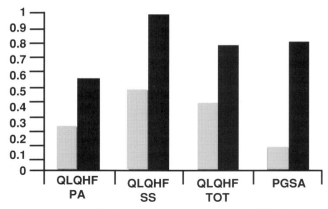

Figure 6.3 Improvement in health-related quality of life in heart failure patients followed up at a nurse-led, outpatient clinic ■ compared to patients with convential follow-up ▨. SS = somatic symptoms. TOT = total. PGSA = patients global self-assessment).

The second randomised trial on the utilisation of a nurse-led, outpatient management programme aimed at identifying the proportion of elderly patients with moderate to severe heart failure eligible for such a programme, examining the applicability of this programme and reasons for its failure; and finally examining the outcome of the programme in a randomised study.[10] The study excluded all patients judged to be in need of specialised care, i.e. those admitted to the department of cardiology. Patients admitted to medical wards, with the exception of those with haematologic and renal diseases, were screened prior to discharge. Patients were included based on clinical criteria for heart failure. Of 1124 patients screened, 158 were included in the study.

The intervention consisted of a structured-care programme based on a nurse-monitored outpatient clinic run in cooperation with the study physicians who were responsible for the instigation of optimal pharmacological treatment. The main goal of the care programme was to teach patients to recognise and monitor symptoms of deterioration and be knowledgeable about the effects and side effects of the medication they had been prescribed. The patients were advised to call the nurse if symptoms worsened or if any questions arose related to their heart failure. Patients were contacted 1 week after discharge and offered a visit to the clinic, together with a relative or a carer. Each patient's care was individually planned and specific goals set up. A specific goal could, for example, be weighing themselves three times a week and knowing what to do in case of weight gain. The patients were provided with a notebook for monitoring daily weight, weekly medication calendars, written guidelines for early recognition of warning signs of clinical problems, and information about when and where to report such symptoms. The nurse contacted patients regularly by telephone with regard to the points raised at clinic visits.

About two-thirds of patients randomised had a measurable ejection fraction and 60% had a value below 40%. The proportion of patients without contraindications to ACE inhibitors who were on or had tried such treatment was 84% and 96% in the usual-care and structured-care groups respectively. The mean follow-up time was 5 months, during which 23 patients never visited the nurse (29%; 95% CI, 19% to 39%). The groups did not differ in the number of readmissions (mean difference 0·1; 95% CI, 0·5 to 0·3), number of days hospitalised, mortality, or survival without readmission.

What could be the explanation for the difference in results in these two studies carried out in the same country? Could it be that the underlying concept behind heart failure outpatient programmes – that skilled monitoring can reduce the rate of subsequent readmission and produce a cost saving above and beyond the cost of staffing the programme – is not valid in Sweden? The experience of similar programmes in other counties has been a reduction in readmission, reduced costs, and improved quality of life.[11]

The results of the first study are in keeping with other similar studies, although the magnitude of the effect varies. This could be attributed to the intensity of the intervention as well as the range of intervention. The study intervention was of medium intensity compared with other studies. It did not, however, include systematic optimisation of drug therapy. One aim was to specifically evaluate the nurse-led intervention independent of any pharmacological effects. Despite this, the patients in the intervention group were receiving ACE inhibitors to a greater extent than in the control group at the end of the 1-year follow-up (75% v 52%, p < 0.05). This could not, however, account for the reduction in readmission since the difference was relatively small and treatment with ACE inhibitors was prescribed successively throughout follow-up.

It has been suggested that the strategy for diuretic adjustment in the later study may not have been optimal.[12] The experience of others is that readmission rates fall when patients monitor their weight daily, regularly see a health-care worker who can assess their jugular venous pressure and hepatojugular reflux test, and are properly advised to adjust their diuretic regimen when fluid retention is demonstrable. Furthermore, it has been commented on that patients requiring specialist care were excluded, but the patients included appeared to be in need of specialist care. It has been demonstrated that patients treated by primary care physicians and internists are not managed in accordance to guidelines to the same extent as those managed by cardiologists, preferably cardiologists specialising in heart failure.[13, 14] Indeed, it was noted that the patients in the study were not treated in accordance with management guidelines for pharmacological therapy.[12]

Are there other factors that could help explain the different results seen in these two Swedish studies? The patients in the first study were about 5 years younger than those in the second study, approximately 75 years and 80 years respectively. In the first study about 50% of patients were women, whereas in the second study only 40% were women. Ejection fractions appeared lower in the first study compared with the second, especially with regard to both the intervention groups, in which they were 31% and 43% respectively. The use of ACE inhibitors and ß-blockers was higher in the second study, which could have to do with an increased use of these drugs over time. Comparing the control groups in the two studies, one could see that in the first study event-free survival was higher and mortality lower, suggesting that the second study included a more severely ill population despite the fact that the ejection fractions suggested the opposite. However, not all patients in the second study had their ejection fraction determined and therefore the mean for those studied may not be representative. All patients in the intervention group in the first study participated and were in contact with the nurse, whereas 29% of patients in the second study never visited the nurse. These differences could, at least partly, explain the difference in outcome.

It would appear, given all the studies suggesting benefit from a nurse-led outpatient clinic, that there are management strategies effective in increasing event-free survival and improving quality of life. However, we feel that both the studies performed in Sweden used an intervention of low intensity. In the first study there were positive effects at 3 months that were attenuated at 1 year. Since the intervention was concentrated to the inclusion phase of the study and was not systematically reinforced, it may have resulted in the diminished efficacy seen at one year. An increased number of visits to the nurse and regular reinforcement of the education programme might have resulted in greater efficacy in the long term. Further studies are needed to confirm the hypothesis behind the use of nurse-led outpatient clinics for heart failure patients in Sweden. Ideally, at least one of these studies should be undertaken at a number of different centres.

Heart failure management in Sweden

Primary care physicians care for most of the patients with heart failure in Sweden. If in need of hospitalisation the majority of patients are treated in wards assigned to general internal medicine. Cardiologists often care for the minority of younger heart failure patients, especially those awaiting heart transplantation and those who have undergone transplantation. In the early 1990s some hospitals with a special interest in heart failure started outpatient clinics for the initiation and titration of captopril therapy. This concept probably arose from the frequency of side effects and adverse events seen in the early era of ACE inhibitor treatment, when large initial doses were used. Since then, much has been learnt about how to use these drugs. Starting with low doses and avoiding dehydration prior to the initiation of therapy has resulted in very few adverse events following initiation of therapy. The early reports on the benefits to be gained by the use of specialised nurses in the management of heart failure patients stimulated further research and development in this area.

In 1997 a survey by way of a questionnaire was performed under the auspices of the Swedish Society of Cardiology (L Erhardt, personal communication). The questionnaire was sent to all existing Swedish hospitals at that time. The aim of the survey was to describe the management of heart failure patients with regard to diagnosis, treatment, and organisational aspects. Of the 90 hospitals that received the survey questionnaire 67 (74%) returned it completed. Ten (15%) of these were university or regional teaching hospitals, 22 (33%) were secondary hospitals, and 35 (52%) were tertiary hospitals.

The extent to which echocardiography was used for the diagnosis of heart failure in outpatients and inpatients was sought. Eight per cent of hospitals used echocardiography for all outpatients with suspected heart failure, whereas 66% used it in most cases, and 26% in selected cases. These figures contrasted with those for inpatients, where 15% used echocardiography in all cases, 73% in most cases, and 12% in selected cases. More than half of the hospitals had no waiting time for an echocardiogram on inpatients, whereas approximately half had a waiting list of 1–4 weeks for outpatients. Almost 60% had access to simplified echocardiography, which has been found to be reliable for the primary evaluation of patients with suspected heart failure.

All university and regional hospitals had nurses specially trained to take care of patients with heart failure, but of all Swedish hospitals only 73% had such nurses (Table 6.1). The same was true for nurse outpatient heart failure clinics: 100% at university hospitals, and 88% and 79% respectively at secondary and tertiary hospitals. In our experience heart failure nurses can become proficient in the titration of heart failure medication (ACE inhibitors, ß-blockers, and diuretics) when given clear directives. As many as 80% of university hospitals, 88% of secondary hospitals, and 52% of tertiary hospitals had delegated the right to adjust doses of the aforementioned drugs to heart failure nurses. Sixty-four per cent of all hospitals had a ward dedicated to heart failure and 60% had specific outpatient heart failure clinics (Table 6.2). Local guidelines or shared care programmes for the management of various illnesses, especially chronic diseases, are relatively common in Sweden. Of all hospitals 60% had local guidelines or a shared care programme. In 82% of these the management programme or guidelines even included primary care. The ultimate responsibility for the care of heart failure patients lay with cardiologists in

78% of hospitals. At the university hospitals it was 100%, at secondary hospitals 90%, and at tertiary hospitals 63%.

Table 6.1 The utilisation of nurses specially trained for the management of heart failure patients in Swedish hospitals.

Type of hospital	Number of hospitals	With heart failure nurses (%)
University/regional	10	100
Secondary	22	73
Tertiary	35	66
All	67	73

Table 6.2 The existence of specific outpatient clinics and wards dedicated to the management of patients with heart failure in Sweden.

Type of hospital	Number of hospitals	With heart failure clinics %	With heart failure wards %
University/regional	10	100	60
Secondary	22	55	77
Tertiary	35	51	57
All	67	60	64

The Swedish cardiac nurses' Working Group for Heart Failure carried out a similar study the following year.[15] They received answers to their questionnaire from 86 hospitals. The aim of the study was to describe nurse-led heart failure care in Sweden. The questionnaire contained questions about the existence of heart failure nurses, their education and delegation, how patient education was provided, presence of a heart failure clinic and if so, how was it organised. Fifty-nine hospitals (69%) had nurses specially trained to take care of heart failure patients – in all 148 nurses. The nurses were involved in patient education including oral and written information, group information (7 hospitals) an educational video (24 hospitals), and an interactive computer-based information program (23 hospitals). Fifty-seven hospitals (66%) had nurse-led clinics that provided follow-up after hospitalisation, telephone counselling, and drug titration. In almost half of the hospitals nurses were authorised to perform specific changes in the doses of diuretics, ACE inhibitors, ß-blockers, and potassium-sparing diuretics.

There is some variation in the data provided in these two surveys on the management of heart failure in Sweden. The results of the survey by Erhardt shows a greater percentage of hospitals with nurse-led clinics, whereas the data from the survey by Strömberg and colleagues has a larger number of hospitals with nurse-led clinics but fewer in percentage terms. One explanation for this could have to do with the larger number of hospitals that did not return the questionnaire in the survey by Erhardt. One would expect hospitals in which nurses were involved in the management of heart failure patients to answer the questionnaire to a greater extent as a reflection of a greater interest in this subject matter. Therefore, as the absolute data suggest, there may have been a substantial increase in the number of nurse-led heart failure clinics in Sweden from 1997 to 1998. In any case, the value of this concept has evidently been accepted despite the paucity of clinical trial data showing efficacy and a Swedish study that suggested a lack of benefit. This may be due to the clinical experience from using this model for the management of heart failure. In our experience the results of this approach are very encouraging both from a health-care provider perspective as well as from a patient perspective. Almost all patients who participated in an evaluation of a management programme for heart failure were very satisfied with the care they received, and felt that the programme should be available for all heart failure patients.[16]

Conclusion

The available data on nurse-led, outpatient heart failure clinics is encouraging. In Sweden, the fast dissemination of this concept and its implementation into clinical practice show that there is a widespread belief in its efficacy. However, there is no consensus on how these clinics should be organised, what training nurses are required to undertake, what patients are most suitable, the responsibility of the nurse in relation to the physician, etc. These questions have to be addressed in the near future. There is also definitely a need for quality control and therefore measures of quality have to be decided on. At present there is widespread interest in the further development of the concept of nurse-led heart failure clinics, which will surely have an important role to play, especially in the implementation of therapeutic guidelines.

References

1   Bergsten-Rydén T, Andersson F. The health care costs of heart failure in Sweden. *J Int Med* 1999; **246**: 275–84.
2   Cline C, Broms K, Willenheimer R, Israelsson B, Erhardt L. Hospitalisation and health care costs due to congestive heart failure in the elderly. *Am J Ger Cardiol* 1996; **5**: 10–23.
3   *Swedish Pharmaceutical Statistics 1998 (Svensk Läkemedelsstatistik 1998)*. Apoteksbolaget AB, Stockholm 1999.
4   Cline CMJ, Willenheimer RB, Erhardt LR, Wiklund I, Israelsson BYA. Health-related quality of life in elderly patients with heart failure. *Scand Cardiovasc J* 1999; **33**: 278–85.
5   Wiklund I, Herlitz J, Hjalmarsson Å. Quality of life five years after myocardial infarction. *Eur Heart J* 1989; **10**: 464–72.

6   Cline CMJ, Björck-Linné AK, Israelsson BYA, Willenheimer RB, Erhardt LR. Non-compliance and knowledge of prescribed medication in elderly patients with heart failure. *Eur J Heart Fail* 1999; **1**: 145-50.

7   Björck-Linné A, Liedholm H, Israelsson B. Effects of systematic education on heart failure patients' knowledge after 6 months. A randomised controlled trial. *Eur J Heart Fail* 1999; **1**: 219–28.

8   Cline CMJ. Heart failure management in the elderly. Thesis, Lund University, Malmö, 1999.

9   Cline CMJ, Israelsson BYA, Willenheimer RB, Broms K, Erhardt LR. Cost effective management programme for heart failure reduces hospitalisation. *Heart* 1998; **80**: 442–6.

10 Ekman I, Andersson B, Ehnfors M, Matejka B, Persson B, Fagerberg B. Feasibility of a nurse-monitored, outpatient-care programme for elderly patients with moderate-to-severe, chronic heart failure. *Eur Heart J* 1998; **19**: 1254–60.

11 Rich MW, Beckham V, Wittenberg C, Leven CL, Freedland KE, Carney RM. A multidisciplinary intervention to prevent the readmission of elderly patients with congestive heart failure. *N Engl Med J* 1995; **333**: 1190–5.

12 Pitt B. Improving outcomes in heart failure. *Eur Heart J* 1998; **19**: 1124–5.

13 Edep ME, Shah ND, Tateoi IM *et al.* Differences between primary care physicians and cardiologists in the management of CHF: relationship to practice guidelines. *J Am Coll Cardiol* 1997; **30**: 518–26.

14 Bello D, Shah NB, Edep ME, Tateo IM, Massie BM. Self-reported differences between cardiologists and heart failure specialists in the management of chronic heart failure. *Am Heart J* 1999; **138**: 100–7.

15 Strömberg A, Martensson J, Fridlund B, Dahlström U. Nurse-led heart failure clinics in Sweden. *Eur Heart J* 1999; **20**: 23.

16 Iwarson A, Cline C, Willenheimer R, Israelsson B, Erhardt L. Congestive heart failure in the elderly: the results of nurse-based patient education and follow-up. *Eur Heart J* 1996; **17**: 290.

7: A specialist nurse-led, home-based intervention in Scotland

LYNDA BLUE, JOHN J V McMURRAY

Chronic heart failure is the most common and the most expensive cause of hospital admission in persons over 65 years of age in the United Kingdom. With an increase in the ageing population this presents a huge public health problem with serious consequences in terms of morbidity, mortality, and health-care expenditure.[1]

Heart failure is a syndrome with a worse prognosis than many common cancers and has a major effect on the lives of patients with severe symptoms.[2] When compared with other chronic illnesses, heart failure has been found to have the greatest negative impact on patient quality of life.[3] Though a number of pharmacological treatments do reduce the morbidity and mortality related to chronic heart failure, the management of this condition remains poor. For example, specialists do not manage the majority of patients.[1] It has recently been suggested that despite well-considered and evidence based guidelines, too few heart failure patients receive treatment of proven efficacy. It could be argued, therefore, that we keep many patients from a longer and better life and increase health-care costs by tolerating "preventable" hospital admissions.[4]

Cleland and colleagues emphasise the need for implementation of what we have learned about heart failure treatment.[5] Many patients have a limited knowledge of both their condition and its treatment;[6] advice on exercise, diet, and immunisation against influenza and pneumococcus is rarely given. As a result of many of these factors a substantial proportion of hospital admissions are thought to be avoidable.[7, 8] For example, studies have shown that approximately 50% of readmissions are potentially preventable through improved patient education, comprehensive discharge planning, and enhanced follow-up.[7, 9] This evidence has led to the suggestion that specialist nurse intervention may be an advantage in these often frail, elderly patients.[10, 11] The main role of the specialist nurse, it is argued, should be to correct these deficiencies in care, outlined more comprehensively by Dr Jaarsma and Professor Dracup in Chapter 2.

It is within this context that this chapter describes the methods, preliminary results, and wider implications of a prospective, randomised, controlled study of a specialist nurse intervention in chronic heart failure in Glasgow, Scotland.

A randomised, controlled study of specialist nurse intervention in chronic heart failure

In undertaking the following study our major objective was to determine whether or not a home-based nurse intervention, used in addition to routine care, can reduce the morbidity and mortality related to chronic heart failure. The participants were patients managed by general physicians (internists) and general practitioners (primary care physicians), who care for the majority of those with chronic heart failure.[1]

Methods

The study was based in the Western Infirmary, Glasgow, in western Scotland. This university-affiliated hospital of approximately 500 beds services the north-west sector of the city of Glasgow: a metropolitan region with approximately 200 000 residents of whom a disproportionate number are elderly and socially disadvantaged, and with higher admission rates compared with the population of Glasgow. Patients were recruited from March 1997 to February 1999. Two specialist nurses with expertise in the management of heart failure were employed to implement the study intervention.

Study endpoints

The primary end-point in this study was time to death or readmission for worsening heart failure. Secondary end-points included all-cause and heart failure-related readmissions, in addition to associated hospital stay. Uniquely for a study of this type, all hospital admissions were classified by a "blinded" end-point committee.

Study patients

All patients admitted on an emergency basis to the acute medical admissions unit in the hospital with a diagnosis of heart failure secondary to left ventricular systolic dysfunction (determined in the majority of cases by echocardiography) were eligible to participate. Patients were excluded, however, if they:

- were unable or unwilling to give informed consent or to comply with the study intervention
- had been admitted with an acute myocardial infarction (unless they had a previous history of chronic heart failure)
- had other life-threatening illness (for example, advanced malignancy)
- were to be discharged to long-term residential care
- resided outside the normal catchment area for the Western Infirmary
- were awaiting cardiac surgery.

Based on these inclusion criteria a total of 165 patients aged between 51–93 years (mean age 75 years), 57% men, were randomised to usual care ($n = 81$) or to the home-based, specialist nurse intervention ($n = 84$). Study follow-up ranged from a minimum of 3 months to a maximum of 12 months (median 9 months).

Usual care

After hospital discharge patients assigned to usual care continued to receive routine management by the admitting physician and, subsequently, their general practitioner. Importantly, the only further contact the specialist heart failure nurses had with the patients in this group was by postal questionnaire to obtain quality of life data. Subsequent hospital admissions and deaths were tracked through the linked hospitalisation and death database for Scotland held by the information and statistics division of the National Health Service in Scotland.

Specialist nurse intervention

Patients randomised to the intervention group continued to have routine care but were also seen by one of two heart failure nurses prior to and after discharge. The main intervention was a series of planned home visits and telephone contact after discharge for a minimum of 3 months and a maximum of 12 months.

Schedule of visits and telephone contact

The first home visit took place within 48 hours of hospital discharge. Subsequent visits were performed at 1 week, 3 weeks, and 6 weeks and then 3, 6, 9, and 12 months after discharge. Scheduled telephone calls were made at 2 weeks and 4 weeks and then at 2, 4, 5, 7, 8, 10, and 11 months. Additional unscheduled home visits and telephone contact could take place as required by the individual patient.

Patients and their families or carers were encouraged to contact the nurses if there was a change in the patient's condition or if there were any problems or questions. The nurses could be contacted Monday to Friday, 0900 to 1700, by mobile telephone. A telephone answering service where patients could leave a message was also provided 24 hours a day, seven days a week. The nurses could also organise general practitioner or hospital clinic visits if it was felt these were indicated.

Telephone contact was an important component of the intervention; the MULTI-FIT research group has demonstrated that a nurse manager, using frequent telephone contact with patients and infrequent telephone contact with cardiologists, can function safely and effectively as a primary mediator of optimal outpatient management of heart failure.[12] A simple telephone call with careful open-ended questions provided the nurse with information about how the patient was coping and whether there were signs or symptoms of clinical deterioration. Most patients and their families and carers valued rapid access to the nurse and reported that it helped reduce anxiety and panic.

Patient record booklet

The patients were provided with a personal record booklet at their first home visit. This provided the nurse's contact telephone numbers, and advice about their condition and its treatment, to encourage self-management. Medication changes, blood pressure, heart rate, weight recordings, and updated biochemistry results were recorded at each home visit. The booklet also provided information for other health-care professionals involved in the patient's management (for example, the patient could take the booklet along to an appointment with the general practitioner or hospital clinic). It was also a valuable tool if the patient needed to call for emergency community-based care or required a hospital admission.

Key components of specialist nurse intervention:

- Assessing patients in their home environment and planning future needs
- Ensuring patients were receiving appropriate therapy in effective doses
- Early adjustment of medication in response to symptoms of clinical deterioration in accordance with prescription guidelines
- Close monitoring of the patient's clinical status and blood chemistry following medication changes
- Providing tailored education, advice, and support about chronic heart failure and its treatment
- Promoting drug and dietary compliance
- Advising patients on life-style changes that would be advantageous to their condition
- Encouraging patients, families, and carers to be actively involved in managing and monitoring their own care
- Being readily available to patients, families, and carers in order to detect and treat early clinical deterioration before symptoms become severe
- Ensuring appropriate and effective communication between the patient, general practitioner, hospital, social services, and all other health professionals involved in the patient's care

---

Main components of the intervention

Whilst it is easy to describe the structure of nurse and patient contacts (see box), it is inherently more difficult to describe how and why an intervention such as this is beneficial to patients. This is not because of an inability to find out which particular component of the intervention is effective, but because there are so many aspects of the intervention that are undoubtedly beneficial. During the implementation of the study intervention the following components appeared to be particularly important.

Assessment

The first home visit by the heart failure nurse specialist was within 48 hours of discharge from hospital, and allowed the nurse to assess:

- how the patient was coping in their home environment
- the patient's chronic heart failure status
- the patient's general health status
- available medical, health-care, and social support
- future health-care needs based upon the above.

This home visit also allowed the nurse to identify how much the patient and the family or carers understood about the condition and its treatment. Many patients feel anxious in the hospital setting, where many learn for the first time that they have heart failure, and are unable to absorb further information. It is usually when the patients return home that they are able to formulate questions about their condition and seek to clarify treatment strategies.

Medication review and adjustment

The nurses reviewed the prescribed medication to ensure patients were receiving appropriate therapy in effective doses. A major component of this particular intervention was the nurses' ability to adjust the patient's medication in accordance with agreed prescription guidelines. These adjustments were made in response to the patient's needs – for example, increasing or decreasing diuretic dosages, and titration of angiotensin-converting enzyme (ACE) inhibitor therapy to achieve the optimal tolerated dose. Furthermore, in suitable patients, ACE inhibitor therapy could be initiated by the nurse following discussion with the general practitioner. Following discussion with the cardiologist and general practitioner, a thiazide diuretic or metolazone was prescribed for a short period for patients who had severe heart failure and were unresponsive to high doses of a loop diuretic.

Close monitoring of blood chemistry

The frequency of blood monitoring was increased for elderly patients in the following circumstances:

- significant changes to the prescribed medication regimen (for example, following changes in the dose of diuretic, initiation or increase in the dose of an ACE inhibitor)
- the presence of clinical instability (for example, if the patient had diarrhoea or vomiting or any upset that might affect renal function)
- patient complaints of symptoms indicative of toxicity (for example, anorexia and nausea, particularly at breakfast time, denoting digoxin toxicity).

Pharmacological education

Education was provided to increase the patients' knowledge about their medication, its action and side effects, and the importance of treatment compliance.

Treatment non-adherence

Non-adherence to prescribed treatment is probably the most common reason for heart failure-related hospitalisation. Over half of all patients significantly fail to adhere to either pharmacological or dietary recommendations.[7, 13] Elderly patients self-adjust their medication regimens for a variety of reasons, primarily lack of knowledge about the expected action of the medication and disillusionment when an immediate and overt improvement of symptoms does not occur.[14, 15] This is of particular concern as older patients often respond unpredictably to prescribed pharmacotherapy owing to a combination of the usual ageing process (affecting, among other things, gastrointestinal absorption, renal function, and hepatic function) and the fact that they have comorbid conditions likely to complicate treatment response further. Some studies do suggest a correlation between improved comprehension of treatment and treatment adherence. Goodyer and colleagues reported the impact of medication counselling in a randomised, controlled trial involving 100 elderly patients with heart failure. Compliance (measured by tablet count) increased from 61% to 93% in the counselled group.[16]

Prescription boxes

Compliance devices were used if the patient was forgetful and/or confused about timing of medication. The patient was issued with the prescription box on a weekly basis. This worked well, although problems arose when the patient's medication was altered and the box had to be immediately returned to the pharmacy for renewal of the updated medication.

Timing of diuretics

Patients were advised about the best times to take their diuretic drugs. Contrary to popular belief, these drugs do not need to be taken at a fixed time of day. In fact, the doses can be timed to suit the patient's daily schedule. As part of this intervention, patients wanting to go out in the morning were advised to take their daily dose when they returned home. However, if a loop diuretic was to be taken late in the day (for example, after 1600–1800 hours) it was pointed out nocturia may result.

Specific education, advice, and support about chronic heart failure

Patients and their families and carers were provided with education, advice, and support about the syndrome of chronic heart failure itself. Importantly, this was tailored to suit their individual needs, and stressed the importance of identifying the early signs and symptoms of worsening heart failure. In the eventuality of such clinical deterioration, clear advice was given about what to do and whom to contact. In this context early adjustment of medication in response to symptoms of deterioration is vital. Michalsen and colleagues point out that despite progressive symptoms patients often do not obtain prompt and adequate treatment and identified that nearly 80% of patients had experienced dyspnoea and oedema for nearly 24 hours before admission.[9] Supporting these data, Friedman and colleagues found that in a group of elderly patients the average duration of acute dyspnoea before hospital admission for chronic heart failure was approximately 24 hours and the duration of oedema and cough 12–14 days.[17] Jaarsma and colleagues found that although a group of chronic heart failure patients in the Netherlands knew what to do when symptoms occurred, they sometimes could not get the attention of a health-care provider in time, or the health-care provider postponed action for a week because of a busy schedule. Changes in the organisation of patient care and the intensity of follow-up are therefore probably essential to prevent unnecessary readmission.[18]

Communication links

If patients required medication changes following hospital discharge there is all too often a discrepancy between the hospital discharge letter and what is documented on the computer in the general practice surgery. As part of the current intervention the heart failure nurse was able to ensure current medication schedules were up-to-date. Many patients were confused by changes in their medication regimen. For example, it was not uncommon to find patients taking their preadmission medication in conjunction with their post-discharge regimen (for example, two different brands of an ACE inhibitor or loop diuretic).

Immunisation

Patients were encouraged to ask their general practitioner for an annual influenza immunisation and a single pneumococcal immunisation. Nichol and colleagues demonstrated a 37% reduction in hospital admissions for deteriorating heart failure among those immunised against influenza during such an outbreak.[19] Opasich and colleagues have also shown, in a group of patients with moderate to severe heart failure, that 23% of episodes of heart failure decompensation were associated with infection; a third of these were pulmonary in origin.[20]

Encouraging self-management and appropriate life-style changes

Patients were encouraged to be actively involved in managing and monitoring their own care and to make any life-style changes that would make a difference to their condition.

Daily weight monitoring

Patients were encouraged to weigh themselves at the optimal time each day on a consistent basis (in the morning after going to the toilet, before breakfast, and before dressing). Patients were asked to record their weight on a provided chart and to report any increase in weight of the order of 1 kg (2lb) or more per day and persisting over more than 2–3 days; this may indicate increasing fluid retention and the need for medication changes. Monitoring weight was also valuable for identifying patients losing too much weight through overdiuresis. Suitable patients were taught to increase their diuretic dosage if they became more breathless or if their weight increased by 1 kg per day and continued to increase on the next day.

Ensuring an adequate supply of medication

Patients were advised to ensure they had an adequate supply of medication, especially at weekends and public holidays, and not to purchase "self-prescribed" medications (such as non-steroidal anti-inflammatory agents) without seeking advice from their nurse or general practitioner.

Fluid intake

Where indicated, patients were advised to restrict their fluid intake to 1500 ml per 24 hours. The nurses provided the patients with a chart showing estimated amounts of fluid in, for example, a cup, mug, or can. Patient co-operation was required.

Management of sodium intake

Patients were encouraged to reduce their salt intake, not to add salt to food at the table, add only a little during cooking, and avoid salty processed foods, cheese, and salty snacks. Unfortunately 75% of salt intake comes from processed foods, and low-sodium food is expensive. To encourage adherence, information was provided to patients on the sodium content of common processed foods. Few modern studies have examined the role of sodium restriction in heart failure. However, excessive sodium retention by the kidneys is known to be a consistent pattern in this condition[21, 22, 23] providing a rationale for restricting sodium intake.

Management of alcohol intake

Patients were advised that alcohol should only be used in small quantities: no more than 2–3 units per day for men and 1–2 units per day for women. Patients whose heart failure was due to alcohol-induced cardiomyopathy were strongly advised to avoid alcohol completely. Cessation of alcohol intake in this group often results in recovery of ventricular function.[24]

General weight management

Patients who were obese were encouraged to lose weight. Reducing obesity will reduce the work of the heart; in addition, it helps lower blood pressure[25, 26] and improve lipid profiles.[27, 28] Patients were encouraged to make gradual changes towards a target loss of around 1 kg per week. Some patients were referred to a group led by a community dietitian or given nutritional counselling by a health professional skilled in weight management and behaviour change. Weight management was aimed at achieving and maintaining a body mass index below 25 kg/m^2.

Cardiac cachexia

Cachexia is a frequent complication of advanced chronic heart failure and involves loss of muscle mass (including cardiac muscle) as well as adipose tissue.[29] Muscle wasting in cardiac cachexia also exacerbates exercise intolerance and enhances the sense of fatigue and dyspnoea. When cachexia was due to nausea or dyspnoea patients were advised to have small, frequent snacks rather than larger, more spaced meals. Oral nutritional (energy) supplementation was also encouraged. Every effort was made to ensure adequate nutrition in these patients. In a study of elderly patients in Sweden, chronic heart failure was the most common single diagnosis in malnourished patients.[30] Further research, to identify strategies to reverse cachexia, is needed.[31]

Smoking advice

Patients were encouraged to stop smoking; the strategies used were tailored to individual patient needs.

Encouraging exercise

Patients in a stable condition were encouraged to increase activities such as walking, cycling, swimming, golfing, and bowling. Quality of life has been shown to be increased following an exercise programme.[32, 33] Whether the effect can be attributed to the exercise or to the additional interest taken in the patient during the trials remains to be decided. However, in other circumstances exercise improves mood probably by the release of endogenous endorphins. The increase in quality of life scores may also be associated with a perceived improvement in breathlessness and a reduction in fatigue.[34]

Follow-up visits

Follow-up visits enabled the nurses to update and reinforce information in any area required, as well as closely monitoring the patient's clinical status and blood chemistry following medication changes and detecting any deterioration in renal function. Appropriate and effective communication was maintained between the patient, general practitioner, carer, hospital, social services, and all health-care professionals involved in the patient's care.

Easy access to the heart failure nurse

It was vital for the nurses to be readily available to patients, families, and carers in order to detect and treat early clinical deterioration before symptoms become severe.

Psychological support

Depression, anxiety, and fear are common in people diagnosed with chronic heart failure.[3, 35] The home visits provided patients, families and carers with psychological support ("someone there") which helped reduce anxiety and panic. There are few published reports about specific programmes of psychological interventions for patients with heart failure. Stewart and colleagues have demonstrated the poor quality of life of these patients compared with those suffering from other chronic diseases.[3]

Preliminary results

A preliminary analysis of the outcome data generated from this randomised study suggests a number of benefits for patients randomised to the nurse intervention during the study.

- There was no difference between the two groups in the number of patients readmitted for any cause; however, there was an approximate

50% reduction in the number of patients admitted for heart failure in the nurse intervention group.

- There was approximately a 25% reduction in the average number of readmissions for any cause, and an approximate 50% reduction in the average number of readmissions for heart failure in the nurse intervention group.
- There was an approximate 50% reduction in the average number of days in hospital for any cause and also in the average number of days in hospital for heart failure in the nurse intervention group.

Discussion

It is well established that in many cases the recurrence of chronic heart failure with the requirement for hospital readmission can be attributed to preventable factors and not to the underlying syndrome itself. This unsatisfactory situation is perpetuated in the UK by a system that undervalues equitable and easy access to health-care professionals, education and the provision of psychological care to help patients with heart failure to make the necessary life-style changes to remain clinically stable as long as possible.

Heart failure is a complicated syndrome to manage. Doctors are often unable to provide optimal heart failure care for these patients owing to budgetary and time constraints, therefore additional or alternative ways of managing these patients are required. The nurse specialist assigned to the care of heart failure patients may become an important co-provider of heart failure care. Without other commitments the nurse specialist may become more experienced in the care of these patients than general practitioners (primary care physicians) and even some cardiologists or internists who lack experience because of their type of practice, and may act as a specialised "safety-net" in case of worsening symptoms. Maintaining a low threshold for contact will enable the specialist nurse to arrange for intervention by specialists at short notice.[4]

The intervention of a specially trained and dedicated nurse can substantially reduce the risk of readmission to hospital in those patients previously hospitalised as an emergency with heart failure.

A study from Adelaide in Australia reported that home-based intervention did not have a statistically significant effect on the number of patients experiencing an unplanned admission or death, but it was effective in preventing individual patients from requiring repeated readmissions with acute heart failure.[11] Previous research had indicated that education and support were effective in improving patients' self-care behaviour, but not sufficiently to decrease readmission.[18]

Key components of the specialist nurse intervention

The key components of this successful nurse intervention appeared to be a combination of:

- regular contact with patients to detect clinical deterioration
- continued adjustment and optimisation of therapy: nurses could initiate changes in medical therapy in accordance to prescription guidelines without medical consultation, which may have resulted in more rapid correction of medical problems such as sodium-volume overload and deteriorating renal function
- educating patients and their families about symptoms of heart failure: how to recognise them at an early stage, what to do, and whom to contact when they occur.

Creating a service

As a result of the apparent beneficial effects of this intervention, the Greater Glasgow Health Board agreed to fund a nurse-led heart failure liaison service (based on the study experience) inaugurated in May 2000. The service aims to optimise the management of patients with chronic heart failure in the community. Specially trained nurses, working in conjunction with general practitioners and hospital physicians, will implement agreed protocols, including medical prescription guidelines, drawn up in conjunction with general practitioners and cardiologists in the city.

Future directions

Nurse-led heart failure clinics

The study described in this chapter was based on home visits only, and was therefore valuable to many of the frail elderly patients who would have otherwise been unable to attend hospital regularly. Developing a nurse-led heart failure clinic in conjunction with home visiting appears to be the most satisfactory way forward. Mobile patients with access to transport could be seen at a clinic, allowing the nurses more time to visit housebound and less well patients. The aim of a heart failure clinic would be to improve the patient's quality of life, promoting drug and dietary compliance, and encouraging self-management through structured follow-up and monitoring, drug titration, and patient education. Erhardt and colleagues have demonstrated that heart failure patients need continuous, long term support outside the hospital environment, so it is mandatory that a system is designed in which patients can be offered optimal care after discharge.[36]

Integrating palliative care

There is no formal support in place for this patient group when palliative management is required. We must recognise that heart failure is a terminal disease. Much has been done for patients with cancer but whilst the network of support for current categories of palliative care patients is highly developed, it has been argued that the needs of those with heart failure have been neglected.[37] Many patients with chronic heart failure underestimate the seriousness of their situation; in a retrospective study of bereaved relatives, only 50% of patients were thought to have known they were dying.[37] Many of these patients had never had either a diagnosis or a prognosis explained to them by their general practitioner or physician. The guidelines drawn up by the Agency for Health Care Policy and Research stress the need to discuss the prognosis with the patient and family.[38] However, many doctors do not do this, and even avoid referring to heart failure at all because patients find it so frightening. Estimating an individual's prognosis is difficult in relation to chronic heart failure but the palliative nature of treatment needs to be discussed with patients if they are to make informed choices about their care and plans for the future.

Conclusions

Our research experience with this type of specialist nurse intervention in heart failure is consistent with that of our international colleagues. There is little doubt therefore, that these types of intervention need to be funded and adopted on a widespread basis. Our current challenge is to establish a successful service of this type in the metropolitan region of Glasgow. We hope that this service will develop into a comprehensive programme for all heart failure patients, regardless of whether they have been admitted to hospital, and incorporate both home visiting and a clinic-based approach to heart failure management. For the first few years, however, we will be concentrating on establishing a strong framework for the service built upon adequate resource funding, a well-developed and defined infrastructure and, most importantly, skilled specialist nurses who can provide high-quality, individualised health care to the heart failure patient.

References

1   McMurray J, McDonagh T, Morrison CE, Dargie HJ. *Eur Heart J* 1993; **14**: 1158–62.
2   Ho KK, Anderson KM, Kannel WB, Grossman W, Levy D. Survival after the onset of congestive heart failure in Framingham Heart Study subjects. *Circulation* 1993; **88**:107–15.
3   Stewart AL, Greenfield S, Hays RD *et al.* Functional status and well-being of patients with chronic conditions. *JAMA* 1989; **262**: 907–13.
4   Balk AHMM. The 'heart failure nurse' to help us close the gap between what we can do and what we can achieve. *Eur Heart J* 1999; **20**: 632–3.
5   Cleland JGF, Swedberg K, Poole-Wilson PA. Successes and failures of current treatment of heart failure. *Lancet* 1998; **352**(suppl. 1): 19–28.

6 Ashton CM. Care of patients with failing hearts: evidence for failures in clinical practice and health services research [editorial; comment] *J Intern Med* 1999; **14**: 138–40.

7 Vinson JM, Rich MW, Sperry JC, Shah AS, McNamara T. Early readmission of elderly patients with congestive heart failure. *J Am Geriatr Soc* 1990; **38**: 1290–5.

8 Chin MH, Goldman L. Factors contributing to the hospitalisation of patients with congestive heart failure. *Am J Pub Health* 1997; **87**: 643–8

9 Michalsen A, Konig G, Thimme W. Preventable causative factors leading to hospital admission. *Heart* 1998; **80**: 437–41.

10 Rich MW, Beckham V, Wittenberg C, Leven CL, Freedland KE, Carney RM. A multidisciplinary intervention to prevent the readmission of elderly patients with congestive heart failure. *N Engl J Med* 1995; **333**: 1190–5.

11 Stewart S, Vandenbroeck AJ, Pearson S, Horowitz JD. Prolonged beneficial effects of a home-based intervention on unplanned readmission and mortality among patients with congestive heart failure. *Arch Intern Med* 1999; **159**: 257–61.

12 West J, Miller NH, Parker KM *et al.* A comprehensive management system for heart failure improves clinical outcomes and reduces medical resource utilization. *Am J Cardiol* 1997; **79**: 58–63.

13 Ghali JK, Kadaia S, Cooper R, Ferlinz J. Precipitating factors leading to decompensation of heart failure. Traits among urban blacks. *Arch Intern Med* 1988; **148**: 2013–16.

14 Cargill JM. Medication compliance in elderly people: Influencing variables and interventions. *J Adv Nurs* 1992; **17**: 422–6.

15 Fineman B, Delice C. A study of medication compliance. *Home Health Nurse* 1992; **10**: 26–9.

16 Goodyer L, Miskelly F, Milligan P. Does encouraging good compliance improve patients' clinical condition in heart failure? *Br J Clin Pract* 1995; **49**: 173–6.

17 Friedman MM. Preadmission symptoms in older adults admitted for heart failure [abstract]. *Circulation* 1995; **92**(suppl. 1): 248.

18 Jaarsma T, Halfens R, Huijer Abu-Saad H *et al.* Effects of education and support on self-care and resource utilization in patients with heart failure. *Eur Heart J* 1999; **20**: 673–82.

19 Nichol KL, Margolis KL, Wuorenma J, Von Sternberg T. The efficacy and cost effectiveness of vaccination against influenza among elderly persons living in the community. *N Engl J Med* 1994; **331**: 778–84.

20 Opasich C, Febo O, Riccardi PG *et al.* Concomitant factors of decompensation in chronic heart failure. *Am J Cardiol* 1996; **78**: 354–7.

21 Packer M. Pathophysiology of chronic heart failure. *Lancet* 1992; **340**: 88–92.

22 Bard KF, Ichikawa I. Pre-renal failure: a deleterious shift from renal compensation to decompensation. *N Engl J Med* 1988; **319**: 623–9.

23 Jacob AJ, McLaren KM, Boon NA. Effects of abstinence on alcoholic heart muscle disease. *Am J Cardiol* 1991; **68**: 805–7.

24 Sonne-holm S, Sorensen TIA, Jensen G, Schnohr P. Independent effects of weight change and attained body weight on prevalence of arterial hypertension in obese and non-obese men. *Br Med J* 1989; **299**: 767–70.

25 Kostis JB, Rosen RC, Cosgrove NM, Shindler DM, Wilson AC. Non-pharmacological therapy improves functional and emotional status in congestive heart failure. *Chest* 1994; **106**: 996–1001.

26 Dattilo AM, Kris-Etherton PM. Effects of weight reduction on blood lipids and lipoproteins: a meta-analysis. *Am J Clin Nutr* 1992; **56**: 320–8.

27 Hankey CR, Rumley A, Lowe GDO, Lean MEJ. Weight loss improves indices of ischaemic heart disease risk. *Proc Nutr Soc* 1995; **54** (2): 94A.

28 Freeman LM, Roubenoff R. The nutrition implications of cardiac cachexia. *Nutr Rev* 1994; **52**: 340–7.

29 Broqvist M, Arnqvist H, Dahlstrom U, Larsson J, Nylander E, Permert J. Nutritional assessment and muscle energy metabolism in severe chronic congestive heart failure: effects of long-term dietary supplementation. *Eur Heart J* 1994; **15**: 1641–50.

30 Scottish Intercollegiate Guidelines Network/Scottish Cancer Therapy Network. *Diagnosis and treatment of heart failure due to left ventricular systolic dysfunction.* Edinburgh: Royal College of Physicians, 1999.

31 Koch M, Douard H, Broustet JP. The benefit of graded physical exercise in chronic heart failure. *Chest* 1992; **101**: 231–5S.

32 Kavanagh T, Myers MG, Baigrie RS, Mertens DJ, Sawyer P, Shephard RJ. Quality of life and cardiorespiratory function in chronic heart failure: effects of 12 months' aerobic training. *Heart* 1996; **76**: 42–9.

33 Coats AJS. Exercise rehabilitation in chronic heart failure. *J Am Coll Cardiol* 1993; **22**: 172–7A.

34 Dracup K. Quality of life in patients with advanced heart failure. *J Heart Lung Transpl* 1992; **11**: 273–9.

35 Erhardt L, Cline C. Heart failure clinics [editorial]. *Heart* 1998; **80**: 428–9.

36 Jones S. Palliative care in terminal cardiac failure [letter]. *Br Med J* 1995; **310**: 805.

37 McCarthy M, Lay M, Addington-Hall J. Dying from heart disease. *J Royal Coll Physicians* 1996; **30**: 325–8.

38 Konstam M, Dracup K, Baker D *et al*. *Heart failure: evaluation and care of patients with left-ventricular systolic dysfunction*. Clinical Practice Guidelines No. 11. AHCPR Publication No. 94-0/612. Rockville, MD: US Department of Health and Human Services, 1994.

8: A specialist nurse-led, multidisciplinary, home-based intervention in Australia

SIMON STEWART, JOHN D HOROWITZ

Like most other industrialised countries, Australia, which has a public health-care system, has to deal with the current limits of response to pharmacotherapy for chronic heart failure. Like our international counterparts, therefore, we have been developing adjunctive non-pharmacological treatment regimens to supplement its standard management. This chapter describes a series of studies examining the potential benefits of a nurse-led, multidisciplinary, home-based intervention for chronic heart failure.

A preliminary study of a nurse-led, multidisciplinary, home-based intervention

In 1995 we undertook a controlled study to determine the effect of a multidisciplinary, home-based intervention on a primary end-point of frequency of unplanned readmission plus out-of-hospital death during 6 months' follow-up among chronically ill cardiac and non-cardiac patients discharged home from acute hospital care.[1]

We recruited 762 chronically ill, medical and surgical patients from the Queen Elizabeth Hospital in Adelaide, a tertiary referral hospital servicing the north-western region of Adelaide, South Australia, and randomised them to either usual care ($n = 381$) or a multidisciplinary, home-based intervention ($n = 381$). The study intervention consisted of counselling of all patients prior to discharge, followed by a single home visit (by a nurse and pharmacist) to patients considered to be at "high risk" of readmission ($n = 314$) in order to:

- optimise the management of prescribed treatment
- identify early clinical deterioration
- intensify follow-up of such patients where appropriate.

During the 6-month follow-up the primary end-point occurred more commonly in the usual-care group (217 v 155 episodes; p < 0.001). Overall, the home-based intervention group demonstrated fewer unplanned readmissions (154 v 197; p < 0.05), out-of-hospital deaths (1 v 20; p < 0.001), total deaths (12 v 29; p < 0.01), visits to the emergency service department (236 v 314; p < 0.001) and total days of hospitalisation (1452 v 1766; p < 0.001). There was a disproportionate reduction in multiple events among study patients (p = 0.035). Hospital-based costs of health care during study follow-up tended to be lower in the intervention group (Au$2190 v Au$2680 per patient). Whilst the cost of implementing the study intervention was Au$190 per patient visited, other community-based health-care costs were similar for both groups.

This nurse-led, multidisciplinary, home-based intervention therefore reduced the frequency of unplanned readmissions plus out-of-hospital deaths within 6 months in a group of older patients with a variety of chronic illnesses. This intervention appeared to be particularly cost-effective in reducing the number of individuals who required multiple admissions to hospital. Moreover, the intervention appeared to have a positive effect on survival.[1]

Subset analysis of chronic heart failure patients participating in the study

The major subclinical group in this preliminary study was patients with chronic heart failure. Considering the apparent beneficial effect of this intervention on recurrent readmissions and possibly survival, we postulated that this intervention would be most cost-effective in this subset of patients. We therefore undertook a post-hoc analysis of these data.

Using the criteria of impaired systolic function, intolerance to exercise, and a history of one or more admissions for acute heart failure, a "high-risk" subset of chronic heart failure patients (n = 97) was selected for further analysis. Of these patients, 49 were randomised to the study intervention and 48 to usual care.[2]

During study follow-up, patients with chronic heart failure assigned to the study intervention had both fewer unplanned readmissions (36 v 63; p < 0.05) and out-of-hospital deaths (1 v 5; not significant). The number of events per patient was 0.76 in the intervention group and 1.4 in the usual-care group (p = 0.03). Study intervention patients also had fewer days of hospitalisation (261 v 452; p < 0.05) and total deaths (6 v 12; not significant). Patients assigned to usual care were more likely to experience three or more readmissions for acute heart failure (p < 0.02). Predictors of unplanned readmission were more days of unplanned readmission during the 6 months prior to study entry, prior admission for acute myocardial ischaemia, and hypoalbuminaemia. Importantly, home-based intervention was also associated with a trend towards reduced risk of unplanned readmission overall.

Overall, therefore, we found that this intervention appeared to be particularly effective in the management of chronic heart failure, with fewer unplanned readmissions and out-of-hospital deaths, and (as with the major cohort) fewer recurrent readmissions.[2] We were, however, unable to demonstrate a definitive reduction in hospital-based costs or mortality among those patients exposed to the study intervention. In order to examine the medium-term effects of the intervention on the original primary end-point, and (more importantly) frequency of recurrent hospital admissions, total hospital stay, cost of hospital-based care, and total mortality, we extended follow-up of all surviving patients for a further 12 months (to a maximum of 18 months after the index hospitalisation).[3]

Results of prolonged follow-up of high-risk patients

During the extended follow-up period, the high-risk heart failure patients assigned to the study intervention continued to accumulate both fewer unplanned readmissions (64 v 125; p < 0.05) and out-of-hospital deaths (2 v 9; p < 0.05), representing 1.4 versus 2.7 events per intervention patient and usual-care patient, respectively (p < 0.05). Patients assigned to the study intervention also had fewer days of hospitalisation (2.5 days v 4.5 days per patient; p < 0.01) and once readmitted, were less likely to experience five or more readmissions (3/31 v 12/39; p < 0.05). Hospital-based costs were significantly lower for intervention patients (Au$5 100 v Au$10 600 per patient; p < 0.05).

Unplanned readmission was independently associated with more days of unplanned readmission within 6 months of study entry. Similarly, a fatal event was independently associated with non-English-speaking status, more days of unplanned readmission in the 6 months before study entry, and a lower left ventricular ejection fraction (LVEF). Conversely, assignment to the study intervention was independently associated with a negative risk of unplanned readmission.

We therefore demonstrated that this intervention was associated with a reduction in unplanned readmissions within 18 months of discharge from acute hospital care in this subset of patients. Once again, it appeared that this intervention was particularly effective in preventing recurrent readmissions to hospital and appeared to have some benefits in respect to more prolonged survival.[3]

A prospective study of nurse-led, multidisciplinary, home-based intervention in chronic heart failure

Based on the results of the preliminary investigation, a study was designed to examine specifically and prospectively a form of this intervention, *modified for individuals with heart failure*, on hospital readmissions and survival among high-risk patients with chronic heart failure recently discharged from acute hospital care.[4]

Methods

Inclusion criteria

Participants were patients admitted to the Queen Elizabeth Hospital in Adelaide under the care of a cardiologist. Chronic heart failure patients were eligible to participate if they were 55 years old or over, were discharged to home, and had been hospitalised at least once with acute heart failure.

Presence of chronic heart failure was defined as both impaired left ventricular systolic function (LVEF 55% or less) and persistent functional impairment indicative of New York Heart Association (NYHA) class II, III, or IV status. Acute heart failure was defined as pulmonary congestion/oedema evident on chest radiography, with a clinical syndrome of acute dyspnoea at rest. Exclusion criteria were extensive, reversible ischaemia precipitating heart failure, valvular heart disease amenable to surgical correction, intended cardiac transplantation, presence of terminal disease, or home address outside the hospital's catchment area.

Study design

A total of 4055 cardiology patients were screened over a period of 14 months commencing March 1997. Of these, 285 patients (7%) fulfilled the clinical criteria for study entry. However, 59 of them (21%) met one or more of the exclusion criteria, and 26 patients (9%) refused to participate or died prior to hospital discharge. A total of 200 patients were therefore recruited and randomly allocated to usual care alone (n = 100) or supplemented by a multidisciplinary, home-based intervention (n = 100).

Immediately prior to hospital discharge patients were interviewed and their medical records reviewed to determine baseline clinical, demographic, and psychosocial characteristics. Specific baseline measures included mental acuity using the Mini-Mental State Examination,[5] functional status using the Katz Activities of Daily Living (ADL) index,[6] and extent of comorbidity using the Charlson index (a cumulative index that adjusts for chronic heart failure and myocardial infarction).[7]

97

Patient management

Usual care

Pre-existing norms for levels of discharge planning were applied to all 200 patients participating in the study without restriction. These included both inpatient and community-based contact with a cardiac rehabilitation nurse, dietitian, social worker, pharmacist, and community nurse where appropriate. All patients had an appointment with their general practitioner and/or the cardiology outpatient clinic within 2 weeks of discharge. In all cases, regular outpatient-based review by the responsible cardiologist was undertaken throughout the follow-up period.

Multidisciplinary, home-based intervention

Patients assigned to the study intervention (n = 100) received, in addition to the same therapy as the usual-care patients, a structured home visit by a qualified cardiac nurse (with post-graduate qualifications in advanced coronary care nursing) 7–14 days following discharge. During this visit the nurse evaluated the patient's clinical progress since discharge, performed a physical examination, and assessed the patient's adherence to the prescribed treatment regimen, understanding of the disease process (including the ability to recognise changes in symptomatic status indicative of worsening heart failure), current level of physical activity, extent of psychosocial support, and pre-existing use of available community-based resources.

On the basis of this comprehensive home assessment, patients and their families (if appropriate) received a combination of remedial counselling, introduction of strategies designed to improve treatment adherence, introduction of a simple exercise regimen, and incremental monitoring by family or carers. If required, patients were referred to their primary care physician for urgent medical treatment. Following the home visit, the cardiac nurse sent a report to the patient's general practitioner and cardiologist detailing both the assessment and any actions taken or recommended. Home visits were repeated only if a patient had two or more unplanned readmissions within 6 months of the index admission. However, all intervention patients were contacted by telephone at 3 months and 6 months to assess their progress and arrange additional follow-up if required, and were encouraged to contact the cardiac nurse if any subsequent problems arose.

Study end-points

Primary end-point

Consistent with previous studies of this type,[2, 8, 9] the primary end-point for the study was the frequency of unplanned readmissions plus out-of-hospital deaths during the minimum 6 months follow-up (the effective duration of study intervention).

Secondary end-points

Other prespecified study end-points were time to first primary end-point (event-free survival) and death, frequency of unplanned readmissions, out-of-hospital deaths, days of unplanned readmission, cost of hospital and community-based health care, functional status and health-related quality of life, and medication-related knowledge within 6 months of the index admission. Unplanned readmission and survival data for the duration of patient follow-up were used to examine the longer-term effects of the intervention.

Data collection

All hospital activity, including associated costs, was monitored through the hospital's medical record and accounting departments. Records of the time and location of all deaths were compiled using the region's birth, deaths and marriages registry. An equal number of patients from each group were randomly selected for evaluation of changes in health-related quality of life and functional status at 3 months and 6 months in comparison with baseline ($n = 68$) using the Australian version of the MOS 36-Item Short-Form Health Survey (SF-36)[10] and the Minnesota Living with Heart Failure questionnaire (MLWHF),[11] and the total cost of community-based health care during the 6 months after the index admission ($n = 66$). Measurement of knowledge of the prescribed cardioactive agents at hospital discharge and then at 1 month and 6 months thereafter, using a previously validated questionnaire for measuring medication-related knowledge,[11] was undertaken for the remainder of patients ($n = 66$). Figure 8.1 summarises the study recruitment and follow-up.

Results

Baseline characteristics

Baseline characteristics. Table 8.1 lists the baseline characteristics of the two groups. Analysis of all baseline data suggested that the groups were well matched for all but number of admissions for acute heart failure and serum creatinine level at hospital discharge. The majority of patients had moderate to severe systolic dysfunction and persistent symptoms despite what would be considered appropriate pharmacotherapy at the time of recruitment. Moreover, as expected, they were generally older and frailer than patients typically recruited to clinical trials.

Table 8.1 Baseline clinical and demographic profile of study cohort.

	Study intervention (n = 100)	Usual care (n = 100)
Demographic profile		
Male	65	59
Mean age (yrs)	75.2 (7.1)	76.1 (9.3)
Live alone	36	32
≤ 8 years formal education	43	47
Congestive heart failure profile		
Median duration of treatment for CHF (months)	21.0 (2.0–42.0)	15.0 (2.0–42.0)
Mean admissions for acute heart failure	2.4 (1.9)	1.9 (1.1)
Mean LVEF [% of patients with a LVEF ≤ 40%]	37 (10) [68%]	37 (11) [60%]
Comorbidity		
Ischaemic heart disease (% with known MI)	77 (79%)	79 (67%)
Chronic airways limitation: Atrial fibrillation	33 : 41	38 : 29
Chronic hypertension: Diabetes	65 : 34	65 : 34
Mean Charlson index score	3.0 (1.5)	3.2 (1.4)
Hospitalisation 6 months before study follow-up		
Mean number of unplanned admissions	1.6 (0.9)	1.7 (1.1)
Median days of unplanned hospitalisation	8.0 (4.0–15.0)	8.0 (4.0–13.0)
Index admission profile		
Mean days of index admission	6.6 (5.8)	6.9 (5.9)
Acute pulmonary oedema at hospital admission	53	51
Mean systolic blood pressure (mmHg)	146 (32)	147 (33)
Acute myocardial ischaemia	18	10
Pharmacotherapy at hospital discharge		
Mean number of prescribed medications	7.6 (2.1)	7.6 (2.1)
Diuretic : nitrate : ACE inhibitor : digoxin	95 : 77 : 75 : 71	98 : 74 : 67 : 60
ß-blocker : warfarin : amiodarone : amlodipine	33 : 28 : 18 : 12	23 : 18 : 15 : 15
Clinical profile at hospital discharge		
Mean sodium concentration (mmol/l)	138 (3.5)	139 (3.2)
Mean creatinine concentration (μmol/l)	0.138 (0.061)	0.165 (0.096)
Mean systolic blood pressure (mmHg)	121 (19)	124 (22)
Sinus rhythm : atrial fibrillation	63 : 31	73 : 25
Mean "dry weight" (kg)	73 (15)	70 (16)
Functional status at hospital discharge		
Dependent for one activity of daily living or more	47	56
Formal home support services	43	47
NYHA class II : III : IV	42 : 46 : 12	48 : 43 : 9
Mean Mini-Mental Score	29.2 (1.8)	28.8 (1.9)

ACE, angiotensin-converting enzyme; CHF, congestive heart failure; LVEF, left ventricular ejection fraction; MI, myocardial infarction; NYHA, New York Heart Association.
Normally distributed continuous data are presented as a mean (± 1 SD). Non-normally distributed continuous variables are presented as a median: IQR, interquartile range.

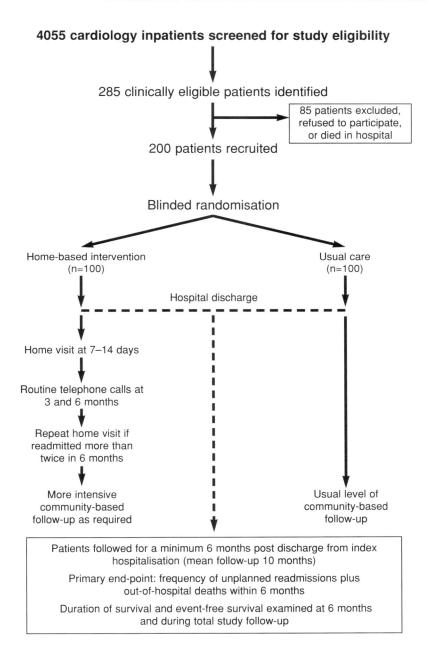

Figure 8.1 Study schema.

Study intervention

A total of 88 of the 100 patients assigned to the study intervention received a home visit: 2 patients died within 48 hours of discharge and 10 patients subsequently refused a home visit despite initial consent. Of 88 initial home visits, 79 (89%) were within the target period of 7–14 days after discharge. The remainder were delayed because of early readmission to hospital. The median duration of these visits was 2 hours (range 1–3.5 hours).

Although the majority of patients were clinically stable at hospital discharge, 35 of the 88 patients visited at home (40%) had one or more signs or symptoms indicative of early clinical deterioration. These included basal crepitations ($n = 19$), a decline in functional status to NYHA class IV ($n = 16$), and onset of decubitus angina ($n = 9$). On the basis of pill counts and self-report, 22 patients (25%) were considered to be clearly non-adherent to their prescribed medication regimen. Similarly, 14 (41%) of the 34 patients prescribed a restricted fluid intake were not adhering to this regimen. Overall, 85 patients (97% of those visited) revealed inadequate understanding of the purpose, effect, and potential adverse effects of their prescribed medication.

Following 33 (38%) of these initial home visits the cardiac nurse contacted the patient's primary care physician or cardiologist in order to arrange immediate review of the patient's clinical status or prescribed treatment. Incremental pharmacist contact was arranged for 19 patients (22%) and new or incremental home-support services for 23 patients (26%) thereafter.

Following the home visits 22 patients (25%) initiated at least one telephone contact with the cardiac nurse in order to clarify issues of concern. In the majority of cases patients were referred to their primary care physician for a non-urgent review, whilst 2 patients described symptoms of acute heart failure and were urgently admitted to hospital. Of the 159 (total) routine telephone contacts made with surviving patients at 3 months and 6 months, only 6 (4%) resulted in immediate referral to the patient's primary care physician. A new home visit was undertaken for 7 of 10 patients who survived two or more unplanned readmissions within 6 months and were not admitted to long-term institutional care thereafter.

Primary end-point

During 6 months of follow-up, patients assigned to the study intervention accumulated a total of 9 out-of-hospital deaths and 68 unplanned readmissions (77 primary events) compared with 11 out-of-hospital deaths and 118 unplanned readmissions (129 primary events) ($p < 0.05$).

Event-free survival

In comparison with usual care, significantly more intervention patients remained event-free at 6 months (51 v 38; $p < 0.05$). Figure 8.2 shows the cumulative probability of event-free survival for the two groups during total duration of patient follow-up (a mean of 10 months). Whilst the two event-free survival curves suggest that the "early" influence of the intervention on the proportion of patients experiencing an event was attenuated beyond 6 months, they also demonstrate that its beneficial effect on the duration of event-free survival (first evident following the implementation of the majority of initial home visits) persisted for up to 9 months. The difference between groups in this respect was significant overall ($p < 0.05$). According to the Cox proportional hazards model, independent predictors of event-free survival were extent of comorbidity as measured by the Charlson index, presence or absence of formal home support services, extent of unplanned hospitalisation in the 6 months before study entry, and study assignment. (Table 8.2).

Table 8.2 Independent correlates of the primary end-point (event-free survival) during 6 months' follow-up according to the Cox-proportional hazards model.

	Unplanned readmission or out-of-hospital death within 6 months			
	No ($n = 89$)	Yes ($n = 111$)	p value	Risk ratio (95% CI)
Mean (SD) Charlson index of comorbidity score	2.6 (1.1)	3.5 (1.5)	< 0.001	1.4 * (1.1, 1.8)
Routine home support services provided following hospital discharge	26 (29%)	64 (58%)	< 0.01	1.9 (1.5, 2.3)
Mean (SD) days of unplanned hospitalisation in the 6 months before study follow-up	8.9 (8.7)	12.8 (12.5)	< 0.01	1.02 † (1.01, 1.04)
Assignment to the multidisciplinary home-based intervention	51 (57%)	49 (44%)	0.03	0.66 (0.53, 0.79)

*, †Where indicated the increased risk of experiencing a primary event is based upon an incremental score of 1 for the Charlson index of comorbidity * and each additional day of unplanned hospitalisation in the 6 months before study follow-up (†).

Unplanned readmission

At 6 months patients assigned to the study intervention had accumulated 68 unplanned readmissions compare with 118 for the usual-care group ($p < 0.05$). The equivalent figures for the extended follow-up period were 118 versus 156 unplanned readmissions ($p = 0.053$). Figure 8.3 shows the accumulated total of unplanned readmissions for the two groups during study follow-up, and demonstrates that beyond 6 months the two groups accumulated a similar number of unplanned readmissions;

essentially maintaining the early trend in favour of the study intervention.

Figure 8.4 shows that the frequency distribution of unplanned readmissions during the 6-month follow-up period was significantly different for the two groups (p < 0.05), with patients assigned to the study intervention both less likely to be readmitted and, if admitted, requiring fewer recurrent (and costly) hospital admissions.

A similar proportion of unplanned readmissions among both groups of patients were associated with a primary diagnosis of acute heart failure; accounting for 34 (50%) versus 58 (49%) of intervention and usual-care readmissions respectively. Recurrent heart failure was also the predominant reason for patients requiring two or more unplanned readmissions. Not surprisingly, the intervention group required fewer days of unplanned hospitalisation, accumulating a total of 460 days versus 1173 days of admission (p < 0.01). Conversely, these patients accumulated more days of elective hospitalization with a total of 87 days versus 25 days of hospitalisation (p = 0.13); the majority of which were for surgical procedures that had been delayed until the patient was considered to be clinically stable. During the entire study follow-up, intervention patients required fewer days of unplanned hospitalisation accumulating a total of 875 days versus 1476 days of admission (p < 0.05).

Mortality

At 6 months a total of 18 intervention patients and 28 usual-care patients had died (p = 0.09). Figure 8.5 represents the cumulative survival curves for the two groups during the entire study follow-up. Although the study intervention appeared to convey an early benefit as regards improved survival, there were no statistically significant differences between groups on the basis of univariate survival analysis. However, the Cox proportional hazards model showed that study assignment was a borderline, independent predictor of survival at 6 months along with duration of the index hospitalisation, left ventricular ejection fraction, and presence or absence of long-term nitrate therapy. (Table 8.3).

Health-care expenditure

As expected, individual health-care costs (in Australian dollars) varied considerably according to the type of health-care resource utilised, with lower overall hospital-based costs among intervention patients ($490 300 v $922 600). Among the subset of patients for whom community-based health-care costs were calculated (n = 66), expenditure per month was similar in both groups ($431 per intervention patient v $438 per usual-care patient). Alternatively, the direct additional cost of the multidisciplinary, home-based intervention was $350 per patient.

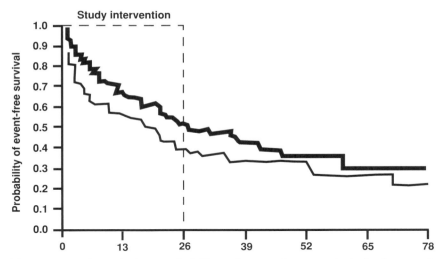

Figure 8.2 Cumulative probability of event-free survival during study follow-up according to study assignment (solid line, intervention group; dashed line, usual-care group).

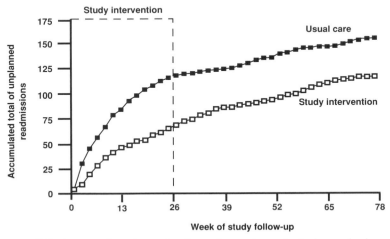

Figure 8.3 Accumulated total of unplanned readmissions during total patient follow-up (open squares, intervention group; solid squares, usual-care group).

Table 8.3 Independent correlates of death during six months follow-up according to the Cox-proportional hazards model.

	Death within 6 months of hospital discharge			
	No (*n* = 154)	Yes (*n* = 46)	p value	Risk ratio (95% CI)
Mean (SD) duration of index admission in days	6.0 (4.5)	9.0 (8.6)	< 0.001	1.07 * (1.04, 1.1)
Mean (SD) left ventricular ejection fraction	38.1 (10.6)	32.8 (10.9)	0.01	0.97 † (0.95, 0.99)
Prescribed long-term nitrate therapy at hospital discharge	110 (71%)	41 (89%)	0.02	3.7 (2.6, 4.8)
Assignment to multidisciplinary home-based intervention	82 (53%)	18 (39%)	0.046	0.54 (0.0, 1.0)

* † Where indicated the risk of dying is based upon each additional day of admission during the index hospitalisation (*) and decrements of 1% in left ventricular ejection fraction (†).

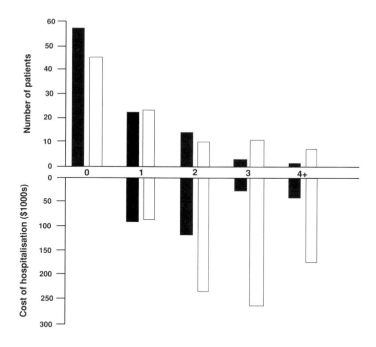

Figure 8.4 Frequency distribution of unplanned readmisions (upper panel) and their cost in Australian dollars (lower panel) during 6 months follow up (solid bars, home-based intervention group; open bars, usual-care group).

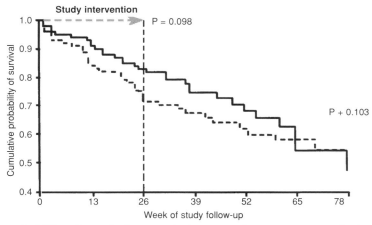

Figure 8.5 The Cumulative survival curves for two groups during the entire study follow-up.

Quality of Life

Table 8.4 summarises the quality of life scores at 3 months and 6 months in comparison with those obtained at the time of initial discharge. There was a general improvement in health-related quality of life over time among surviving patients. However, although the two groups had similar baseline scores, among surviving patients at 3 months (62 of 68), patients assigned to the study intervention had significantly improved scores as measured by the physical component sections of the SF-36 and the MLWHF. Among surviving patients at 6 months, however, scores were similar for both groups.

Table 8.4 Changes in health-related quality of life scores at 3 and 6 months compared to baseline among surviving patients.

Health-related quality of life measure	Study intervention	Usual care	p value
Baseline scores	(n = 34)	(n = 34)	
Baseline MLWHF score	65 (47, 70)	62 (49, 73)	0.36
Baseline SF-36 physical health component score (%)	26 (21, 32)	23 (18, 28)	0.19
Baseline SF-36 mental health component score (%)	58 (48,76)	56 (37, 68)	0.71
Scores at 3 months (comparison with baseline)	(n = 32)	(n = 30)	
∂ MLWHF score	−19 (−41, 1)	−1 (−29, 10)	0.04
∂ SF-36 physical health component score (%)	16 (5, 27)	3 (−8, 14)	0.02
∂ SF-36 mental health component score (%)	10 (−19, 19)	5.7 (−9, 31)	0.48
Scores at 6 months (comparison to 3 months)	(n = 29)	(n = 24)	
∂ MLWHF score	−17 (−35, -8)	− 12 (−35, −8)	0.30
∂ SF-36 physical health component score (%)	17 (3, 27)	16 (3, 31)	0.53
∂ SF-36 mental health component score (%)	7 (−15, 31)	19 (10, 31)	0.46

All scores are presented as a median (IQR). Higher scores from the Minnesota Living with Heart Failure (MLWHF) questionnaire (comprising 21 questions and a score range of 0–105) indicate reduced quality of life, and therefore *negative* changes in score denotes improvement. Conversely, lower scores from the MOS 36-Item Short-Form Health Survey (SF-36) indicate impaired quality of life and *positive* changes in score denote improvement (physical and mental health component scores are averaged from 3 and 5 items respectively, scores range from 0% to 100%).

Study implications

The results of this controlled study suggest that a relatively inexpensive, specialist nurse-led intervention augments the efficacy of pharmacotherapy in limiting readmission to hospital and death in a group of patients with severe, chronic heart failure over a period of at least 6 months. It represents the first time that a non-pharmacological intervention of this type has been reported to both prolong event-free survival and reduce hospital use among patients with chronic heart failure discharged from acute hospital care.

Characteristics of the study cohort

Consistent with recently reported studies of hospitalised heart failure patients,[7, 11-34] the majority of whom are not suitable for cardiac transplantation, this was a typically older and inherently frail cohort of patients. Readmission and survival rates for usual-care patients were similar to those reported from larger-scale studies of heart failure patients. For example 54% (95% CI, 44% to 64%) of patients assigned to usual-care had an unplanned readmission within 6 months of the index hospitalisation, and 35% (95% CI, 26% to 45%) had died within 12 months. These figures are entirely consistent with the studies reported by Krumholz et al.[8] and Jaagosild et al.[12] who demonstrated that in relatively unselected cohorts of older patients with chronic heart failure, approximately half of patients are readmitted within 6 months and a third of them are dead within a year following an acute hospitalisation. Only 50% of unplanned readmissions were precipitated by worsening heart failure; this reflects the high prevalence of multiple chronic disease states in this patient group and possibly also the increased risk of development of adverse effects of pharmacotherapy in such individuals.[35]

Potential benefits of this type of intervention

The generally poorer health outcomes among this type of patient, whilst reflecting the limited therapeutic impact of current pharmacological agents, provide an impetus for the development of adjunctive non-pharmacological treatment regimens. In this context a number of multifaceted strategies designed to address those factors associated with clinical instability among chronic heart failure patients have been evaluated in a limited number of randomised[10, 13, 31] and non-randomised[36-39] studies. Overall, these studies suggest that strategies incorporating home visits and nurse-mediated, multidisciplinary intervention are likely to be superior to purely hospital-based strategies[40, 41] in respect to limiting hospital use among patients with chronic heart failure.

Comparison with other studies

In view of differences in major end-points and relatively small sample sizes, it is potentially misleading to compare the extent of associated benefit in the current study with those of other studies of this type. Nevertheless, available data suggest that this type of intervention is at least as effective in reducing admissions over comparable follow-up periods as those utilised in previous studies. For example, in the key study of a nurse-directed, multidisciplinary intervention Rich *et al.* reported that 54% versus 64% of usual-care patients and intervention patients respectively were event-free, and 16% versus 6% respectively had accumulated two or fewer unplanned readmissions at 90 days.[13] In the current study the equivalent 90-day figures were 57% versus 71% and 15% versus 8%. Moreover, the approximate 60% reduction in days of unplanned hospitalisation at 6 months in the current study is consistent with the magnitude of beneficial effect we have observed previously,[10] and is comparable with the magnitude of effect of the successful interventions examined by Rich *et al.*[13] and by Cline et al.[31] at 3 months and 12 months respectively.

Cost implications

This type of intervention appears to be particularly effective in reducing the number of patients who require frequent and costly unplanned readmissions. The cost of the intervention, and the increased community-based health-care services it initially engendered, were more than compensated for by the savings associated with the reduction in hospital stay compared with usual care. Because of the variability of hospital-based costs within the total cohort, the difference between groups did not reach statistical significance. At the very least, however, we have demonstrated that the reduction in hospital use associated with the intervention has the potential to offset the cost of its implementation, and is unlikely to be associated – in the medium term at least – with greater hospital use among surviving patients.

Possible mechanisms of beneficial effect

Whilst it is inherently difficult to identify exact mechanisms of beneficial effect of multifaceted interventions of this type, we postulated that home visits represent the most effective component of this type of intervention. In the current study, therefore, all patients were subject to the same level of discharge planning. Moreover, considering the association between both non-specialist management and inappropriate pharmacotherapy with poorer health outcomes,[7, 42-48] all study patients were managed by a cardiologist and received treatment appropriate to current guidelines.[49] We also postulated that the major benefit of visiting patients with heart failure in the home following acute hospitalisation would be derived from a better assessment of the patients' management of their illness and a more accurate determination of their future needs. In this respect we found that approximately one-third of patients had signs of early clinical deterioration likely to lead to rehospitalisation without remedial intervention. A post-hoc analysis was performed to determine the independent predictors of "non-fatal", early clinical deterioration among the 88 patients in whom it could be reliably measured (therefore excluding the 10 patients who refused a home visit) using multiple logistic regression; as before, entry of variables into the model occurred at a univariate significance level of 0.05 and backward, stepwise rejection of variables thereafter at the 0.05 level of significance. Early clinical deterioration was defined as either death, unplanned readmission, or clinical deterioration detected at the home visit within 14 days of discharge. On initial univariate analysis, nine baseline parameters were found to be significantly associated with early clinical deterioration in this cohort of 88 intervention patients. These included age, left ventricular ejection fraction, serum creatinine and urea levels at hospital discharge, comorbid burden as determined by the Charlson index, extent of activities of daily living as determined by the Katz ADL score, amiodarone therapy at hospital discharge, presence or absence of chronic airway limitation, and presence or absence of diabetes (type 1 or type 2). On subsequent multivariate analysis there were only two independent determinants of early clinical deterioration: greater age (p = 0.008, odds ratio 1.1 per year; 95% CI, 1.03 to 1.2), and greater comorbidity as determined by the Charlson index (P < 0.001, OR 2.0 per unit score of 1; 95% CI, 1.4 to 2.9).

Consistent with previous data suggesting that this type of intervention is associated with improved treatment compliance[34] and fewer medication-related admissions,[33] the home visit resulted in a more accurate determination of extent of adherence to prescribed treatment and the implementation of strategies designed to optimise treatment thereafter. Whilst Jaarsma and colleagues failed to show a significant reduction in hospital readmissions in a similar cohort of patients after a home visit by a cardiac nurse, during which time they provided additional education and counselling, they did show that such an intervention was associated with an increased preparedness of patients to care for themselves.[50] Consistent with these data, intervention patients demonstrated a greater understanding of their medications shortly following the home visit.

Follow-up data suggested that the two groups did not begin to diverge in respect to the primary end-point until the initial home visits were implemented. The combination of telephone follow-up and repeat home visits thereafter enabled the cardiac nurse to monitor the success of the initial home visit and adjust implemented strategies accordingly. Multivariate analysis demonstrated that the beneficial effects of the intervention were independent of baseline clinical and demographic parameters (including those for which the two groups were found to be significantly different).

Residual issues and study caveats

With advances in the pharmacological treatment of chronic heart failure (for example, more extensive use of ß-adrenoceptor antagonists[3, 4]), it is possible that the apparent incremental benefits of applying this type of intervention may be reduced. However, hospitalised heart failure patients are frequently intolerant of a complex pharmacological regimen. Moreover, greater number of medications and associated adjustments in dosage increase the probability of both non-compliance and development of adverse effects.[33] It is also possible that the applicability of this intervention may be limited overall. However, although the current investigation was performed at a single institution the results are consistent both with those of our preliminary investigations[10, 25] and those performed in the USA[13, 36, 38] and Europe.[31, 37] Moreover, preventable hospital readmissions are a phenomenon common to nearly all developed countries.[51]

Conclusion

In this series of studies we showed that a specialist nurse-led, multidisciplinary intervention has the potential to significantly improve health outcomes in individuals with severe, chronic heart failure. Importantly, this type of intervention improves patient care and subsequent health outcomes whilst reducing overall health-care costs. It therefore represents an attractive adjunct to the current management of chronic heart failure and may well prove to be useful in the management of other chronic cardiac disease states associated with frequent hospital use.

References

1   The SOLVD Investigators. Effect of enalapril on survival in patients with reduced left ventricular ejection fractions and congestive heart failure. *N Engl J Med* 1991; **325**: 293–302.
2   The CONSENSUS Trial Study Group. Effects of enalapril on mortality in severe congestive heart failure: results of the Cooperative North Scandinavian Enalapril Survival Study (CONSENSUS). *N Engl J Med* 1987; **316**: 1429–35.
3   The Australia-New Zealand Heart Failure Research Collaborative Group. Effects of carvedilol, a vasodilator beta-blocker, in patients with congestive heart failure due to ischemic heart disease. *Circulation* 1995; **92**: 212–18.
4   Packer M, Bristow M, Cohn J *et al*. The effect of carvedilol on morbidity and mortality in patients with chronic heart failure. *N Engl J Med* 1996; **334**: 1349–55.
5   Gorkin L, Norvell NK, Rosen RC *et al*. Assessment of quality of life as observed from the baseline data of the studies of left ventricular dysfunction (SOLVD) trial quality-of-life substudy. *Am J Cardiol* 1993; **71**: 1069–73.

6   Rector TS, Kubo SH, Cohn JN. Validity of the Minnesota Living with Heart Failure Questionnaire as a measure of therapeutic response to enalapril or placebo. *Am J Cardiol* 1993; **71**: 1106–7.

7   Reis SE, Holubkov R, Edmundowicz D *et al.* Treatment of patients admitted to hospital with congestive heart failure: specialty-related disparities in practice patterns and outcomes. *J Am Coll Cardiol* 1997; **30**: 733–8.

8   Krumholtz HM, Parent EM, Tu N *et al.* Readmission after hospitalization for congestive heart failure among medicare beneficiaries. *Arch Intern Med* 1997; **157**: 99-104.

9   Burns RB, McCarthy EP, Moskowitz MA, Ash A, Kane RL, Finch M. Outcomes for older men and women with congestive heart failure. *J Am Geriatr Soc* 1997; **45**: 276–80.

10   Stewart S, Pearson S, Horowitz JD. Effects of a home-based intervention among patients with chronic congestive heart failure. *Arch Intern Med* 1998; **158**: 1067–72.

11   Lowe J, Candlish P, Henry D, Wlodarcyk J, Heller R, Fletcher P. Management and outcomes of congestive heart failure: a prospective study of hospitalised patients. *Med J Aust* 1998; **168**: 115–18.

12   Jaagosild P, Dawson N, Thomas C *et al.* Outcomes of acute exacerbation of severe congestive heart failure. *Arch Intern Med* 1998; **158**: 1081–9.

13   Rich MW, Beckham V, Wittenberg C, Leven CL, Freedland KE, Carney RM. A multidisciplinary intervention to prevent the readmission of elderly patients with congestive heart failure. *N Engl J Med* 1995; **333**: 1190–5.

14   McMurray J, Hart W, Rhodes G. An evaluation of the cost of heart failure to the National Health Service in the UK. *Br J Med Econ* 1993; **6**: 99–110.

15   O'Connell J, Bristow M. Economic impact of heart failure in the United States: time for a different approach. *J Heart Lung Transplant* 1993; **13**: S107–12.

16   Rich MW, Freedland KE. Effect of DRG's on three-month readmission rate of geriatric patients with congestive heart failure. *Am J Publ Health* 1988; **78**: 680–4.

17   Wolinsky F, Smith D, Stump T, Overhage J, Lubitz R. The sequale of hospitalization for congestive heart failure among older adults. *J Am Geriatr Soc* 1997; **45**: 558–63.

18   Vinson JM, Rich MW, Sperry JC, Shah AS, McNamara T. Early readmission of elderly patients with congestive heart failure. *J Am Geriatr Soc* 1990; **38**: 1290–5.

19   Gooding J, Jette AM. Hospital readmissions among the elderly. *J Am Geriatr Soc* 1985; **33**: 595–601.

20   McDermott M, Feinglass J, Lee P *et al.* Systolic function, readmission rates, and survival among consecutively hospitalized patients with congestive heart failure. *Am Heart J* 1997; **134**: 728–36.

21   Rich MW. Epidemiology, pathophysiology, and etiology of congestive heart failure in older adults. *J Am Geriatr Soc* 1997; **45**: 968–74.

22   Croft JB, Giles WH, Pollard RA, Casper ML, Anda RF, Livengood JR. National trends in the initial hospitalization for heart failure. *J Am Geriatr Soc* 1997; **45**: 270–5.

23   Ghali J, Cooper R, Ford E. Trends in hospitalization rates for heart failure in the United States, 1973-1986. *Arch Intern Med* 1990; **150**: 769–73.

24   McMurray J, McDonagh T, Morrison CE, Dargie HJ. Trends in hospitalization for heart failure in Scotland 1980-1990. *Eur Heart J* 1993; **14**: 1158–62.

25   Stewart S, Pearson S, Luke CG, Horowitz JD. Effects of a home based intervention on unplanned readmissions and out-of-hospital deaths. *J Am Geriatr Soc* 1998; **46**: 174–80.

26   Stewart S, Vandenbroek A, Pearson S, Horowitz J. Prolonged beneficial effects of a home-based intervention on unplanned readmissions and mortality among congestive heart failure patients. *Arch Intern Med* 1999; **159**: 257–61.

27   Stewart S, Marley JE, Horowitz JD. Effects of a multidisciplinary, home-based intervention on unplanned readmissions and survival among patients with chronic congestive heart failure: a randomised controlled study. *Lancet* 1999; **354**: 1077–83.

28   Folstein M, Folstein S, McHugh P. Mini-Mental State. A practical method for grading the cognitive state of patients for the clinician. *J Psych Res* 1975; **12**: 189–98.

29   Katz S, Ford A, Moskowitz R, Jackson B, Jaffe M. The index of ADL: a standardized measure of biological and pyschosocial function. *JAMA* 1963; **185**: 914–19.

30   Charlson ME, Pompei P, Ales KL, McKenzie RC. a new method of classifying prognostic comorbidity in longitudinal studies: development and validation. *J Chron Dis* 1987; **40**: 373–83.

31 Cline C, Israelsson B, Willenheimer R et al. A cost effective management programme for heart failure reduces hospitalisation. Heart 1998; 80: 442–6.

32 Ware J, Sherbourne C. The MOS 36-item short-form health survey (SF-36): conceptual framework and item selection. Med Care 1992; 30: 473–83.

33 Stewart S, Pearson S. Uncovering a multitude of sins: medication management in the home post acute hospitalisation among the chronically ill. Aust NZ J Med 1999; 29: 220–7.

34 Rich MW, Gray DB, Beckham V, Wittenberg C, Luther P. Effect of a multi-disciplinary intervention on medication compliance in elderly patients with congestive heart failure. Am J Med 1996; 101: 270–6.

35 MacDowall P, Kaira P, O'Donoghue D, Waldek S, Mamtora H, Brown K. Risk of morbidity from renovascular disease in elderly patients with congestive cardiac failure. Lancet 1998; 352: 13–16.

36 West J, Miller N, Parker K, Senneca D et al. A comprehensive management system for heart failure improves clinical outcomes and reduces medical resource utilization. Am J Cardiol 1997; 79: 58–63.

37 Kornowski R, Zeeli D, Averbuch M et al. Intensive home-care surveillance prevents hospitalization and improves morbidity rates among elderly patients with severe congestive heart failure. Am Heart J 1995; 129: 162–6.

38 Fonarow GC, Stevenson LW, Walden JA et al. Impact of a comprehensive heart failure management program on hospital readmissions and functional status of patients with advanced heart failure. J Am Coll Cardiol 1997; 30: 725–32.

39 Hanumanthu S, Butler J, Chomsky D et al. Effect of a heart failure program on hospitalization frequency and exercise tolerance. Circulation 1997; 96: 2842–8.

40 Weinberger M, Oddone EZ, Henderson WG. Does increased access to primary care reduce hospital readmissions? N Engl J Med 1996; 334: 1441–7.

41 Naylor M, Brooten D, Jones R, Lavizzo-Mourey R, Mezey M, Pauley M. Comprehensive discharge planning for the hospitalized elderly. Ann Intern Med 1994; 120: 999–1006.

42 McDermott M, Lee P, Mehta S, Gheorghiade M. Patterns of angiotensin-converting enzyme inhibitor prescriptions, educational interventions, and outcomes among hospitalized patients with heart failure. Clin Cardiol 1998; 21: 261–8.

43 Luzier A, Forrest A, Adelman M, Hawari F, Schentag J, Izzo J. Impact of angiotensin-converting enzyme inhibitor underdosing on rehospitalization rates in congestive heart failure. Am J Cardiol 1998; 82: 465–9.

44 Pearson TA, Peters TD. The treatment gap in coronary artery disease and heart failure: community standards and the post-discharge patient. Am J Cardiol 1997; 80: 45–52H.

45 Smith N, Psaty B, Pitt B, Garg R, Gottdiener J, Heckbert S. Temporal patterns in the medical treatment of congestive heart failure with angiotensin-converting enzyme inhibitors in older adults, 1989 through 1995. Arch Intern Med 1998; 158: 1081–98.

46 Stafford RS, Saglam D, Blumenthal D. National Patterns of angiotensin-converting enzyme inhibitor use in congestive heart failure. Arch Intern Med 1997; 157: 2460–4.

47 Edep ME, Shah NB, Tateo IM, Massie BM. Difference between primary care physicians and cardiologists in management of congestive heart failure: relation to practice guidelines. J Am Coll Cardiol 1997; 30: 518–26.

48 Ghali J, Giles T, Gonzales M et al. Patterns of physician use of angiotensin converting enzyme inhibitors in the inpatient treatment of congestive heart failure. J La State Med Soc 1997; 149: 474–84.

49 The ACC/AHA Task Force on Practice Guidelines (Committee on Evaluation and Management of Heart Failure). Guidelines for the evaluation and management of heart failure. J Am Coll Cardiol 1995; 26: 1376–98.

50 Jaarsma T, Halfens R, Huijer Abu-Saad H et al. Effects of education and support on self-care and resource utilization in patients with heart failure. Eur Heart J 1999; 20: 673–82.

51 Michalsen A, König G, Thimme W. Preventable causative factors leading to hospital admission with decompensated heart failure. Heart 1998; 80: 437–41.

9: Key components of specialist nurse-led programmes in chronic heart failure

SIMON STEWART, LYNDA BLUE

Before describing how best to establish a specialist nurse programme in chronic heart failure, this brief chapter summarises what we consider are the key components of this type of intervention. Importantly, the components are relevant to both home and clinic-based interventions. Because these components are often interrelated, they are presented in no particular order. We suggest that the following list should be used in the preliminary stages of planning a service to ensure that it evolves into an effective one. We would also suggest that this list be considered in conjunction with the range of expert opinions offered in the other chapters.

Key components of specialist nurse interventions in heart failure

A qualified specialist nurse who can effectively manage heart failure patients

The specialist nursing staff are the key component of this type of intervention. Without appropriate training, remuneration, and support, this may be the hardest component to reproduce on a consistent basis. Ideally, the specialist nurse will be experienced in managing heart failure, have the ability to work independently, and, display initiative, as well as engendering trust and respect from both the patient and other health-care professionals.

Identifying high-risk patients

Although specialist nurse-led interventions are undoubtedly effective in optimising the overall management of heart failure, they have proved to be most cost-effective in optimising the management of high-risk patients (those most at risk of recurrent hospitalisation). Whilst all hospitalised heart failure patients should be considered to be at high risk, not all require intensive intervention. It is probably more cost-effective, therefore, to provide a "safety-net" of minimal intervention to all hospitalised heart failure patients and provide incremental care to those who need it most. This requires well-defined protocols for assessing patients and deciding upon the level of care they require.

A holistic approach

Reflective of the inherent nature and intent of nursing practice, and the many complex problems older heart failure patients typically encounter, it is important that the patient's health care is managed within a holistic framework.

Interdisciplinary collaboration

The heart failure patient typically requires the advice and expertise of a number of healthcare professionals. However, in many cases the potential value of such health care is thwarted by the haphazard manner in which it is delivered. Specialist nurses, if properly trained and trusted, are able to assess the individual needs of the patient and co-ordinate their care without interfering with the professional integrity and practice of other health-care professionals involved. Certainly, without the nurse's ability to refer patients to other members of the healthcare team (for example, cardiologist, general practitioner, and community pharmacist) on a reliable basis – if necessary, urgently – there is little doubt that these types of intervention would prove to be largely ineffective.

Optimising pharmacological therapy

A consistent feature of this type of intervention is a mechanism by which the patient's prescribed pharmacological regimen is optimised, the patient's overall ability to manage the pharmacotherapy is assessed, and any problems addressed. In some health-care systems it may be possible to empower the specialist nurse to alter the pharmacological regimen using strict, evidence based protocols and the close support of an experienced physician (for example, a cardiologist). If this is not feasible, it is important that the specialist nurse is able to initiate action when it is required (for example, referral to the general practitioner or community pharmacist).

Individualised health care

Although it is easy to recommend individualised care, achieving this within a modern health-care system is difficult. However, wherever possible the assessment and support of the heart failure patient should be tailored to the needs of the patient (for example, introducing a flexible diuretic regimen).

Continuous monitoring of high-risk individuals

Patients who are most at risk of clinical deterioration or factors that can precipitate such deterioration must be monitored on a consistent basis.

Care for the patient's immediate family or carers

In many instances intervention is most effective when it addresses the needs of the patient's family and carers (for example, improving their understanding of heart failure and its treatment, or arranging for respite care).

Easy access to the specialist nurse

Patients often wait too long before seeking care when faced with worsening symptoms. In many cases, clinical deterioration or anxiety-related symptoms may be alleviated by an unscheduled call to the specialist nurse who has an intimate knowledge of the patient's health status and problems and is able to offer timely advice or intervention. In practice, patients and their families often appreciate the ability to quickly contact the specialist nurse and clarify issues of concern with someone they know and trust.

Expert support

It is unlikely that any intervention of this type will be successfully established without the support of senior nurses, cardiologists, and community-based physicians. In terms of optimising the patient's pharmacological regimen, more tangible support is often required. Conversely, in terms of the referral and overall management of patients, more tacit support is required.

Evidence based approach

Applying an evidence based approach to the patient's management (for example, the pharmacological regimen) reduces the scope for criticism and opposition to this type of intervention.

Facilitation of self-management

Despite the ability to offer incremental support, the specialist nurse should always strive to facilitate more effective self-management. For example, patients should be encouraged to weigh themselves daily if required and alter their diuretic therapy accordingly. Providing an information booklet facilitates self-management.

Education

Educating patients and their families to manage heart failure more effectively is a challenging, but essential component of this type of intervention. Theorists suggest that adults learn best when they perceive a need (and are therefore motivated) and are both physiologically and psychologically stable – a situation that is rarely found in the hospital setting. In many cases it is more appropriate to educate the family or carers rather than the patient, and it is important that the educational programme is flexible using a number of approaches (for example, written material, video and audiotapes, and counselling). Essential topics include the causes and chronic nature of heart failure, and how to manage heart failure on a day-to-day basis.

Psychosocial support

Although the effectiveness of psychosocial support is difficult to measure, and therefore hard to justify, it represents one of the cornerstones of any intervention of this type. Ideally, the extent of such support should reflect the individual needs of the patient and the family. Formal assessment of the patient in respect to extent of anxiety and depression in addition to quality of life represents a good foundation for evaluating such needs.

Discouraging hospital admissions

A natural consequence of incremental patient assessment is the discovery of more health problems and situations in which it appears likely that the patient requires hospitalisation. However, the inherent risks – contracting a nosocomial infection, for example, or physiological and psychological disorientation during hospitalisation – must be considered carefully before patients are admitted to hospital. Except in emergencies, the specialist nurse should not have to make the decision whether the patient should be hospitalised. Consulting a third party (the patient's general practitioner or cardiologist) minimises the risk of unnecessary hospitalisations and helps to maintain a consistent "admission threshold".

Interpreting

Patients who are unable to communicate effectively with health-care professionals because of a language barrier are at particular risk of poorer health outcomes. Wherever possible these patients should be offered the opportunity to communicate with the specialist nurse in their own language using a qualified interpreter.

Detecting clinical deterioration

Clearly, the optimal time to address clinical deterioration is almost immediately after it occurs. However, this rarely happens. Many patients are hospitalised or die without hospitalisation, simply because they did not seek help immediately, or recognise that their condition required treatment. It is important, therefore, that the patient is assessed on a regular basis (especially in the first few weeks following acute hospitalisation). Patients should also be able to attract health care immediately. Probably most importantly, patients (or their families) should be taught to recognise the times when they should seek advice or treatment.

Conclusion

As discussed in Chapter 3, the evidence supporting this type of intervention appears to be convincing. However, there is little information to guide the transition from research into practice – hence this book. To increase the likelihood of a specialist nurse-led heart failure service reaching its full potential and improving health outcomes, we would recommend that all of the above components be considered carefully. This applies equally to a clinic-based or home-based approach. The next chapter provides a step-by-step guide to implementing a specialist nurse-led service, incorporating all the components mentioned above.

10: Establishing a specialist nurse-led service

SIMON STEWART, LYNDA BLUE

Putting research into practice is never easy. The fact that specialist nurse-led interventions are designed to optimise the interaction between patients, their complex treatments, and the often unwieldy health-care system in which they are managed, makes the task of establishing such a programme a difficult one. This chapter describes, in detail, the process by which a successful programme of this type can be established.

It should first be acknowledged that we have an inherent bias towards establishing programmes that involve a large component of home-based intervention, as this has been the focus of our own research efforts (see Chapters 7 and 8). Moreover, the information provided here, is largely influenced by our experiences in establishing a specialist nurse service for heart failure patients in Glasgow. However, we have attempted to set out the principles of establishing such a service, rather than prescribing how it should operate. As described in Chapters 5 and 6, there is certainly a place for a clinic-based approach. Indeed, given sufficient funding we would gladly operate a specialist nurse-led service for the post-discharge management of heart failure using a combination of home-based and clinic-based follow-up. The process of establishing a service is presented as a series of steps. In the spirit of the development of this type of intervention, however, we strongly recommend a healthy dose of critical thought in considering both the advice given and the order in which the steps are presented.

Choosing the right kind of approach

Chapter 3 provided an overview of the evidence for implementing specialist nurse-led interventions to optimise the post-discharge management of chronic heart failure. This information was supplemented by more comprehensive reports from an international panel of researchers from Australia, New Zealand, Scotland, Sweden, and the USA. Clearly there are a number of possible forms of specialist nurse-led interventions, and the following points should be carefully considered:

- What are the limitations of the current health-care system?
- What is the most practical means by which health outcomes can be improved?

The research undertaken by Ekman and colleagues in Sweden represents a good example of a considered approach to the dilemma of selecting the appropriate type of intervention.[1] They found that a clinic-based approach was not suitable for all of their heart failure patients because of the time and effort required to attend the clinic itself. They therefore recommended that a home-based approach be adopted.

Step 1: Develop a precise description of the service with a list of aims and objectives

Before introducing a service of this type it is important to establish a strong framework upon which it can be built. Having chosen the type of service you wish to implement, it is helpful to provide a concise description of the service and its aims and objectives to the large number of administrators and health-care professionals who are affected by its implementation (see box).

Step 2: Establish formal links with other relevant health-care services

One of the most important considerations in establishing this type of service is where the specialist nurse will be based. There are, of course, advantages and disadvantages associated with any decision made in this regard. For example, locating the specialist nurse in the hospital setting will facilitate the screening and recruitment of patients to the service and hopefully increase access to hospital-based professionals (including cardiologists) and services (biochemistry, haematology, and echocardiography). On the other hand, nurses based in the hospital may become physically or professionally isolated from community-based health-care professionals, including the patient's primary care physician. Although it is the most difficult option, it is best if the specialist nurse is incorporated into the culture of both the hospital and community-based services. This undoubtedly requires prominence in both settings; at least in the initial stages of service development, and at regular intervals thereafter.

In order to ensure the long-term viability of the service, both formal and informal links need to be forged. Following is an example of the type of formal arrangement required to establish this kind of service (home-based in this instance).

Framework for employment of a specialist nurse in chronic heart failure

Principal employer (community-based role)

The specialist nurse will be employed by the primary care organisation. This position will involve the following essential roles:

- management of the patient with chronic heart failure in the community in conjunction with the patient's general practitioner and cardiologist
- development of links with other community services, including community-based nurses, health visitors, community-based pharmacists, social services, palliative and emergency care services.

Secondary employer (hospital role)

In addition to the above, the specialist nurse will also be based at the acute-care hospital servicing that particular community, in an honorary position allowing full access to hospital records and services. This position will encompass the following essential roles:
- identifying hospitalised patients with chronic heart failure who meet the criteria for post-discharge specialist nurse management
- promoting the service with staff in whatever speciality or general units chronic heart failure patients are usually managed (medical, cardiology, coronary care, and geriatric units).
- liaising with ward staff regarding patient referral to the service and timing of discharge from hospital
- accessing cardiology expertise for advice and clinical support
- developing links with other important services (echocardiography, biochemistry, haematology, pharmacy, cardiac rehabilitation, and palliative care).

Step 3: Select the type of patient to be eligible for intervention

Ideally, the criteria used to select patients will be as inclusive as possible and therefore incorporate few exclusion criteria. However, when establishing a service it is inherently practical to fine-tune established procedures and protocols (and perhaps more importantly, the skills of any newly appointed specialist nurses) by concentrating on patients whose management is relatively

Description of a specialist nurse-led service for chronic heart failure patients

This service aims to optimise the management of patients with chronic heart failure in the community. Specially trained nurses will work with both hospital and community-based health-care professionals to achieve this goal. The nurses will implement agreed protocols, including medical prescription guidelines, drawn up in conjunction with leading general practitioners (primary care physicians) and cardiologists in the region. All protocols will be reviewed and approved by the appropriate authorising bodies.

Aims of the service
- To improve the post-discharge management of patients with chronic heart failure
- To improve the quality of life of patients with chronic heart failure
- To avoid unnecessary hospital readmissions
- To provide seamless care between primary and secondary care

Patient-specific objectives
- To assess patients in their home environment and plan for their future needs in accordance with the service guidelines
- To review the prescribed medication regimen to ensure that patients receive appropriate pharmacotherapy in effective doses.
- To work to agreed prescription guidelines drawn up in conjunction with general practitioners and cardiologists
- To monitor the patient's clinical status and blood chemistry following medication changes
- To ensure appropriate and effective communication between the patient, general practitioner, carer, ambulance services, hospital, social services, and all other health-care professionals involved in the patient's care
- To provide patients, families, and carers with tailored education, advice, and support
- To act as a resource for other health-care professionals involved with the patient.
- To advise the patient on life-style changes that would be advantageous to their health
- To encourage patients (and their family or carers as appropriate) to be actively involved in managing and monitoring their own care
- To provide easy access for patients, family, and carers to contact the specialist nurse in order to detect and treat early clinical deterioration before symptoms become severe

Service-specific objectives
- To ensure that the overall nursing and medical care provided keeps pace with research evidence (for example, effect of telemonitoring systems)
- To monitor, evaluate, and audit the service at regular intervals to ensure both a high standard of care and the effectiveness of the service as a whole in improving health outcomes.
- To facilitate effective links with other health-care services relevant to the care of the patient with chronic heart failure (including palliative care services)

straightforward using well-established guidelines (especially those relating to medical treatment). For example, it would be more advisable to manage patients with chronic heart failure secondary to left ventricular systolic dysfunction rather than those with diastolic dysfunction or primary valvular dysfunction. Unfortunately, it may prove impractical to restrict patients according to comorbidity likely to complicate treatment (for example, concurrent renal and respiratory illness) because these conditions are so common in older patients with chronic heart failure. Following is an example of the criteria that can be used to recruit patients to this kind of service.

Criteria for admission to the service

Inclusion criteria

Patients must have a documented diagnosis of chronic heart failure and have had at least one emergency hospital admission related to worsening heart failure. Heart failure must be caused by left ventricular systolic dysfunction (as determined by echocardiography, radionuclide ventriculography, or coronary angiography). Patients must be discharged to home and reside within the hospital's catchment area.

Exclusion criteria

Patients will be excluded on the following basis:

- unwillingness to receive the additional support
- impaired cognitive ability determined by the Mini-Mental State test[2]
- major communication problems
- other life-threatening illness requiring palliative care (advanced malignancy).

When initiating the service it is probably better to increase the number of patients gradually to allow teething problems to emerge and be managed in a controlled manner. If, for example, many patients require an interpreter, it may be advisable initially to restrict their numbers. Managing the patients across a communication barrier further complicates an already complex situation – please see Step 9 for specific advice on dealing with such patients.

Step 4: Establish a concise protocol for admitting patients to the service

In many ways the most difficult process is identifying and "capturing" *all* eligible patients. This requires a team approach within the hospital from which patients are recruited. Although the specialist nurse is probably the best-qualified person to screen all admitted patients, screening is a time-consuming process and would leave little time for the nurse to do anything else. Clearly, therefore, there needs to be a mechanism by which eligible patients are identified and referred to the specialist nurse for possible intervention.

Creating a partnership with hospital staff

In the initial stages of developing a new service it is especially important to spend time explaining exactly what will be happening and why the service will be of benefit to members of the health-care system who are affected by it. For hospital-based health professionals who come into contact with potential candidates for the new service, it should be openly acknowledged that their workload will be (initially at least) increased. However, by assisting the specialist nurse to identify and refer eligible patients for the service, and then gather appropriate information and ensure appropriate discharge planning, they are likely to reduce their workload in the longer term. In the first few months of the service, therefore, the specialist nurse needs to spend a good deal of time creating a partnership with hospital staff – becoming "part of the furniture". When this partnership is firmly cemented it should be possible to implement the following type of protocol for identifying and recruiting patients.

Identifying eligible patients during their hospitalisation

Senior nurses or treating medical officers will screen all patients admitted to the hospital for heart failure and alert the specialist heart failure nurse to their presence. A paging system is useful for rapid notification and to allow appropriate scheduling of the nurse's timetable – the earlier the notification, the better. Once notified of a potential candidate for the service, the heart failure nurse will undertake the following steps.

1 Review the patient's medical and nursing records to document the following information:

- extent of left ventricular systolic dysfunction (for example, echocardiograph reports)
- duration of chronic heart failure (for example, date of first diagnosis).
- number of previous admissions for heart failure
- other active medical and social problems
- contributing factors related to the current hospitalisation (for example, arrhythmia, deteriorating renal function, or treatment non-adherence).

2 If the patient appears to be eligible but does not have a recent measurement of left ventricular function, arrange for an echocardiogram to be performed and obtain a copy of the report in order to determine final eligibility.
3 Definitively determine whether the patient is eligible for the service in accordance with the inclusion and exclusion criteria.

Initial contact with the patient

Once an eligible patient is identified the heart failure nurse will approach the patient (and family if appropriate), describe the offered service and ascertain whether they are willing to receive the additional support. *This is particularly important when offering a service with a significant component of home-based intervention.*

Baseline assessment

If the patient is a willing recipient of the service it is important to perform a baseline evaluation as follows.

- If appropriate, assess the patient's mental status using an abbreviated mental test (for example, the Mini-Mental State test).
- Document the patient's baseline details, relevant medical history, admission medication and other active medical and social problems in the heart failure nursing records.
- Document in the patient's medical and nursing notes the date the patient was assessed, and whether the patient is to be followed up with the support of this service.

Specific actions prior to patient discharge

Once a patient has been admitted to the service it is important to know the date of discharge. This requires close liaison with the hospital staff – in particular medical and nursing personnel. With the ever-increasing pressure to reduce duration of hospital stay during the life of the service, this will no doubt become increasingly difficult. Nevertheless, to help prevent early readmission and to optimise post-discharge care, the heart failure nurse may need to request additional admission time for higher-risk individuals (see below) in order to guarantee that either a home visit or a clinic appointment is implemented shortly following hospital discharge. In any case, immediately before hospital discharge the heart failure nurse should:

- review the patient's medical and nursing records for any relevant developments

- record in the specialist nurse's specific case records the patient's discharge medication; biochemistry, blood pressure, heart rate, weight, New York Heart Association (NYHA) classification, and whether or not oedema is present
- obtain a copy of the patient's discharge medication from pharmacy
- arrange the date and time of the first home visit and/or clinic appointment
- provide the patient with a telephone number for emergency contact
- update all information in the heart failure nursing records and database
- issue the patient with an information and record booklet (see below) which will provide the patient with a contact telephone number.

Step 5: Establish precise operational guidelines for the service following patient discharge

Creating a harmonious relationship with community-based services

The principles that were used to ensure a harmonious relationship with hospital staff and services should be applied to developing the relationship with the community-based health-care professionals, although the diversity of these health workers will make this more difficult to achieve. Once again, however, it is important to identify who will be most affected by the service and to convince them that it will be of overall benefit to them and, most importantly, to the patient. The most important healthcare professional to consider is the general practitioner. Dealing with these healthcare professionals on an organisational level helps to spread the broader message and provides information about the service; but in order to attain a trusting and an effective relationship, it is advisable to take the time on an individual level to inform and clarify points of issue with each patient's community-based physician: another good reason for gradually building up the service.

Having strict guidelines and protocols that are agreed upon by the major stakeholders and specifying the exact role of the specialist heart failure nurse will facilitate this process. The following represents an example of specific guidelines for a home-based service.

Post-discharge care

Immediately following the patient's discharge from hospital the heart failure nurse will send a letter to the patient's general practitioner and any other health-care professional involved in the community-based care, detailing both the hospital treatment and the patients enrolment into the service.

First home visit

Within 72 hours of the patient's discharge from hospital the specialist nurse will visit the patient at home and perform the following assessments as appropriate (Figure 10.1):

- assess the patient's heart failure status (for example, NYHA class, oedema and sleeping pattern)
- assess the patient's general health status
- identify the available medical, nursing, and social support systems
- review the patient's medication to ensure they are receiving appropriate therapy in effective doses and adjust it according to medical therapy guidelines
- document the prescribed medication in the patient-held record booklet
- check and record the patient's blood pressure, heart rate, and weight
- check the blood chemistry
- update the patient's record booklet
- assess how much the patient understands about their condition and its treatment
- assess the patients adherence to prescribed treatment
- update and reinforce the patient or carer with any information required
- provide additional educational support designed to increase the patient's knowledge of the prescribed medication (for example, the purpose, dosage, and potential side effects)
- ensure the patient has an adequate supply of medication
- educate the patient about daily weighing (for example, in the morning after going to the toilet, before having breakfast, and before getting dressed)
- provide additional education and advice concerning:
  - diet (including sodium intake, fluid intake, alcohol intake, weight reduction)
  - smoking
  - exercise
- advise the patient to have an annual influenza and single pneumococcal immunisation
- encourage the patient and the family or carers to be actively involved in managing and monitoring their own care
- plan the patient's future needs in accordance to the service guidelines and medical therapy guidelines
- communicate appropriate and effective information to all other health professionals involved in the patient's care.

Underlying the above process is the need to ensure an accurate determination of the patient's health-care and psychosocial needs. Using the assessment made in the home (and this also applies to a clinic-based approach), the specialist nurse should be able to determine, in consultation

127

with the patient, the family, and other important health-care professionals, the optimal level of monitoring, treatment, and support required to maintain clinical equilibrium.

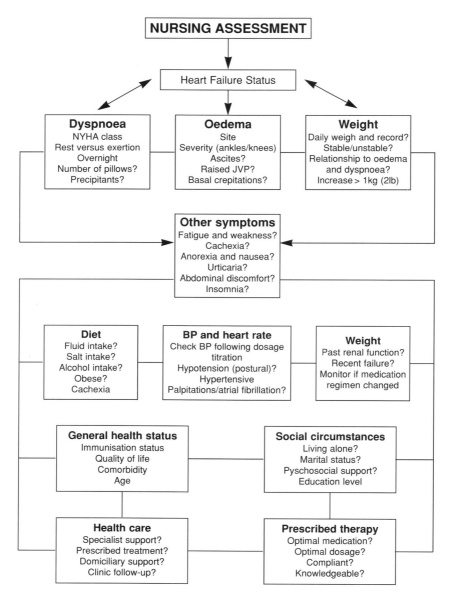

Figure 10.1 Nursing assessment of heart failure – the many factors to consider.

Step 6: Establish precise operational guidelines for patient follow-up

One of the greatest areas of uncertainty concerning this type of intervention is exactly what level of follow-up – whether home-based, clinic-based, or a combination of both – should be implemented. In Chapter 3 it was argued that this type of intervention would be most effective when incorporating a multidimensional approach to the complex interaction between patients, their treatment, and the health-care system. This almost undoubtedly means that some patients will be exposed to a component of intervention that is either unhelpful to them personally or is not particularly effective. Similarly, it is unlikely that we will ever prescribe a "universal" dose of this type of intervention and achieve the same outcomes. Probably the best approach is to provide a "safety-net" or core programme of intervention for patients enrolled into the service and then base the frequency and intensity of follow-up thereafter on established protocols for assessing patients according to individual need.

The following protocol represents a flexible regimen of home-based nurse–patient contact founded on the principles of recognising those at high risk and the need for continuous monitoring and assessment.

Purpose of follow-up home visits

Follow-up home visits should be tailored to the individual's needs in accordance with the service and medical therapy guidelines. The heart failure nurse will:

- continue to adjust and optimise medical therapy where indicated according to established guidelines
- monitor the patient's blood chemistry closely, particularly if there is evidence of biochemical instability and deteriorating symptoms, or if changes to the medication regimen have been made (monitoring as per medical therapy protocol).

Assessment criteria and schedule of follow-up nurse contact

Minimum service

Regardless of their risk profile, all patients (and their family and carers where appropriate) enrolled in the service will be offered the following:

- a home visit within 72 hours of discharge to assess them in the home environment.
- a second home visit 2–4 weeks after hospital discharge
- telephone contact at 3 months and every 3 months thereafter

- the ability to contact the specialist heart failure nurse in case of any problems or clinical deterioration
- the right to be redirected to the heart failure nurse service at any time
- to receive the above if they require a subsequent unplanned readmission to hospital.

Incremental intervention according to risk

Based on the following four components of assessment, patients will receive either the minimum amount of intervention or a more intensive and prolonged programme of follow-up.

Symptomatic status

Patients can be (arbitrarily) divided into those who are symptom-free and those in whom symptoms persist following hospital discharge. In both of these groups there will be patients who are either at "low" or "high" risk for future events such as unplanned readmission or even death without hospitalisation.

Appropriateness of treatment

Regardless of an individual's symptoms, treatment will be either *appropriate* or *inappropriate*.

Risk status

Patients can be considered to be at either high or low risk of future events on the following basis.

Low-risk patients are:

- knowledgeable about their condition and treatment
- compliant with medication and diet
- receiving adequate social support
- not in need of changes.

High-risk patients have:

- a poor understanding of their condition and its treatment
- a history of recurrent admissions for heart failure
- poor compliance with medication and diet
- inadequate social support
- an unsuitable lifestyle.

Intensity and frequency of intervention

Using the above criteria, patients can be categorised as follows, with the intensity and frequency of care modulated accordingly.

Group 1 (symptom-free)

(A) Low risk and appropriately treated

For patients at low risk and appropriately treated regular home visiting is unlikely to have much benefit, and telephone contact on an infrequent basis (for example, 3 monthly) is all that is required. These patients will be encouraged to make non-scheduled telephone contact should their condition deteriorate. These patients will therefore receive the "minimum service" unless their condition or risk profile subsequently changes.

(B) Low risk but inappropriately treated

In this group of patients the main aim is to optimise the patient's medication in accordance with the agreed medication guidelines (monitoring medication changes and blood chemistry). Patients will be visited weekly until the medication regimen is appropriate and their blood chemistry is stable. Telephone contact should be made 1 week later; if the patient remains stable subsequent telephone contact is only required on an infrequent basis (for example, 3 monthly). These patients will be encouraged to make non-scheduled telephone contact should their condition deteriorate.

(C) High risk but appropriately treated

In high-risk, appropriately treated patients, intervention is aimed at improving the patient's understanding of the condition and its treatment, and where indicated increasing social support. The patient should be visited weekly until modifiable risk factors are fully addressed, in accordance with the patient's needs and wishes (usually no more than four home visits will be required). Monthly telephone calls will be made until all correctable issues are resolved. Patients will also be encouraged to make non-scheduled telephone contact should their condition deteriorate. A home visit will be made at 3 months.

(D) High risk and inappropriately treated

The intervention in high-risk patients who are appropriately treated is aimed at improving the patient's understanding of the condition and its treatment; where indicated, increasing social support; and optimising the patient's medication in accordance with the agreed medication guidelines. Visits should be weekly until the patient is compliant with an appropriate medication regimen and modifiable risk factors have been fully addressed, in accordance with the patient's needs and wishes (usually no more than four home visits will be required). Monthly telephone calls will be made thereafter until all modifiable issues are resolved. Patients will also be encouraged to make non-scheduled telephone contact should their condition deteriorate. A home visit will be made at 3 months.

Group 2 (symptomatic)

(A) Low risk and appropriately treated.

One of the objectives of intervention in low-risk appropriately treated patients is, where possible, to adjust what is already considered to be appropriate therapy to improve the patient's clinical status and to minimise any adverse effects of treatment. This will involve application of the medication guidelines and appropriate monitoring of any therapeutic changes implemented (including blood chemistry). The patient *may* require a number of home visits if there is scope for symptoms to improve. *It must be acknowledged, however, that it may not be possible to resolve symptoms completely in all patients and therefore further adjustment of treatment may be inappropriate.* However, the patient is also likely to benefit from other components of this type of intervention. The second objective, therefore, is to provide additional support to individuals who remain symptomatic despite optimal therapy but who would, for example, benefit from psychological support. On this basis, further home visits may be warranted, followed by regular telephone follow-up thereafter. Patients will also be encouraged to make non-scheduled telephone contact should their condition deteriorate. A home visit will be made at 3 months.

(B) Low risk but inappropriately treated

The purpose of the intervention in this group of patients is to adjust their therapy to improve clinical status and minimise adverse effects, by application of the medication guidelines and appropriate monitoring of any therapeutic changes implemented (including blood chemistry). Patients will require home visits until symptoms improve and the patient is compliant with an appropriate regimen. A scheduled telephone call is made 1 week later; if the patient is stable, telephone contact is continued monthly thereafter as long as this is felt to be required. *It may not be possible to resolve symptoms completely in all patients even after appropriate treatment is implemented.* Patients will also be encouraged to make non-scheduled telephone contact should their condition deteriorate. A home visit will be made at 3 months.

(C) High risk but appropriately treated

The object of intervention in high risk patients who are appropriately treated is to adjust therapy to improve symptoms and signs and to minimise the potential for adverse effects. This will involve application of medication guidelines and appropriate monitoring of any therapeutic changes implemented (including blood chemistry). Patients will require home visits until symptoms have improved and risk factors are fully addressed in accordance with the patient's needs and wishes (usually no more than four home visits will be required in relation to risk factors). Telephone contact monthly should be made thereafter as long as this is felt to be required. *It may not be possible to resolve symptoms completely in all patients.* Patients will also be encouraged to make non-scheduled telephone contact should their condition deteriorate. A home visit will be made at 3 months.

(D) High risk and inappropriately treated

The object of intervention in inappropriately treated, high-risk patients is to adjust therapy to improve the patient's clinical status and minimise any adverse effects of treatment, by application of the medication guidelines and appropriate monitoring of any therapeutic changes implemented (including blood chemistry). Patients will require weekly home visits until they are compliant with an appropriate medication regimen, their symptoms have improved, and modifiable risk factors have been fully addressed in accordance with the patient's needs and wishes (usually no more than four visits will be required in relation to risk factors). Telephone contact should be maintained at monthly intervals as appropriate thereafter. Once again, it should be remembered that it may not be possible to resolve symptoms completely in all patients. Patients will also be encouraged to make non-scheduled telephone contact should their condition deteriorate. A home visit will be made at 3 months.

Table 10.1 is a schedule of home-based intervention based on the above groups. It should be noted, once again, that clinic-based visits can be substituted for home visits and that the same principles for altering the frequency and intensity of the intervention based on the patient profile and immediate needs apply.

Step 7: Auditing the service

The negative result of the trial of increased access to primary care reported by Weinberger and colleagues is a salient reminder that an intervention of this type, like any other medical or nursing "treatment", has the potential to lead to negative outcomes.[3] Despite the increasing evidence supporting specialist nurse-led interventions in heart failure, it is imperative that the newly created service is audited to ensure that health outcomes have improved. After a reasonable amount of time for the service to become properly organised and for the correct guidelines and protocols to be implemented, regular, independent auditing of the service's effectiveness should be instituted. The auditing process should evaluate the service from a number of perspectives, including the following.

Health-care utilisation

A major aim of the service should be to reduce rehospitalisation rates. Ideally, all rehospitalisation occurring among those admitted to the recruiting hospital with a diagnosis of chronic heart failure (regardless of whether the patient was exposed to the service or not) should be monitored. If possible, rehospitalisation rates (over at least 6–12 months) should be compared with a previous period (for example, compared with a previous calendar year) and then compared with a cumulative basis thereafter. These comparisons can be made on an overall basis (all heart failure patients) and on the basis of exposure or non-exposure to the intervention. Making any comparison on this basis and with other hospitals is problematic without consideration of influencing variables other than the syndrome itself (for example, age, deprivation, comorbidity, and level of health care). The cost of these admissions should also be calculated.

Table 10.1 Schema for applying a specialist nurse-led service in heart failure.

	Group 1 (Symptom-free)				Group 2 (Symptomatic)			
	A	B	C	D	A	B	C	D
Low risk	✔	✔			✔	✔		
Appropriately treated	✔		✔		✔		✔	
High risk			✔	✔			✔	✔
Inappropriately treated		✔		✔		✔		✔
Initial home visit within 72 hours	✔	✔	✔	✔	✔	✔	✔	✔
Second home visit at 2–4 weeks	✔	✔	✔	✔	✔	✔	✔	✔
Routine 3 monthly phone-calls	✔	✔	✔	✔	✔	✔	✔	✔
Weekly home visits for the first month		✔	✔	✔	✔	✔	✔	✔
Weekly home visits extended for up to 1–2 months								✔
Weekly phone calls to reassess status				✔		✔	✔	✔
Monthly phone calls to reassess health status			✔		✔			
Re-evaluation if readmitted with repeat of at least one home visit	✔	✔	✔	✔	✔	✔	✔	✔

Key points
- All patients will be subject to the "safety-net" of at least two home visits plus 3-monthly phone calls.
- Patients will be regularly reassessed and the amount of follow-up increased or reduced based on their clinical and psychosocial status.
- The specialist heart failure nurse will work towards maximising the impact of the intervention and limiting contact thereafter (excepting patient-initiated phone calls).
- The management of patients who are either symptomatic and/or receiving inappropriate treatment after 3 months will be reviewed by the specialist heart failure nurse co-ordinating the service in consultation with the cardiologist and general practitioner.

Patient satisfaction and quality of life

Whilst hospitalisation rates are important, it is equally important to ensure that the intervention is making a positive impact on patients' quality of life and satisfaction with their health care. A number of tools for measuring quality of life (both specific to heart failure and related to general health status) have been described in previous chapters. Ideally, both of types of questionnaire should be used to measure changes in the patient's quality of life, with additional consideration of their NYHA class. It is not necessary to audit every patient but to generate a random sample from which measurements can be made. Measuring satisfaction with health care is much more problematic on a formal basis. It is possible, however, on an informal basis (for example, with a few well-directed questions) to gather useful information – as long as the mode of auditing is appropriate to the patient (for example, verbal questioning for older patients), allows for candid responses, and is performed on an independent basis.

Family and carer satisfaction and quality of life

Although family and carers are frequently identified as vital cogs in the management of heart failure, they are often overlooked when the burden of heart failure is measured. While an intervention may improve the quality of life of the individual with heart failure, it is possible that people caring for that individual may be adversely affected by the fact that they have little or no respite from that burden of care. Moreover, they may be asked to take a greater role than before; something that may be too onerous for an older partner, for example, who also suffers from chronic illness. Family and carers should therefore always be included in the auditing process.

Hospital-based health professionals

A new service may increase the workload of certain hospital staff (for example, nursing staff) and through resentment and lack of commitment the process of identifying patients and preparing them for discharge may be subsequently undermined. Such problems may only come to light during confidential auditing. In order to maintain goodwill it is imperative that any identified problems are quickly resolved with the assistance and involvement of hospital staff.

Community-based health professionals

It is imperative that community-based healthcare professionals are given the opportunity to air grievances and suggest possible improvements to the service. Our own experiences suggest that cardiologists and general practitioners or primary care physicians feel extremely threatened by the introduction of this type of intervention, but that given time they come to appreciate the service and even provide constructive advice.

Step 8: Appointing and training personnel

The key to successful intervention is the experience and expertise of the specialist nurse. Without the appointment of nurses who are highly motivated, and who have demonstrated expertise in the management of heart failure and the ability to use their own initiative, the service will probably fail to reach its full potential. In order to select the right personnel, it is important to attract high-quality candidates by offering a generous salary package as well as the opportunity to perform in an innovative and rewarding role, and then applying a rigorous selection process.

Number of personnel required

In practical terms it is likely that one nurse will be able to manage 200 heart failure patients per annum being discharged from a single hospital. However, this does not account for holidays and sick leave and the additional staff who consequently need to be employed on an ad-hoc basis. It is undoubtedly more economical to consider a large-scale service encompassing a number of hospitals within a well-defined region. For example, it would be more advisable to appoint one full-time equivalent nurse per 100 000 population (approximately) and a regional co-ordinator who is able to act in a combined role of senior adviser, educator, administrator, auditor, mediator, and clinician (with a limited patient workload).

Essential qualifications

At the very least, potential candidates for the position of specialist nurse in heart failure should fit the following profile:

- professionally qualified as a nurse (for example, Registered Nurse)
- at least 5 years' experience overall
- at least 2 years of recent cardiology experience
- excellent communication skills
- experience in working in an autonomous position
- a proven ability to work effectively in a multidisciplinary setting
- some computing skills
- driving licence.

Additional qualifications

At interview, the following attributes should be used to assess the candidates on a more definitive basis:

- previous community-based nursing experience
- specific expertise in managing patients with heart failure
- further qualifications (for example, Critical Care Certificate) and/or higher nursing qualifications (master's degree)
- experience in research or auditing
- advanced information technology skills.

Selecting a co-ordinator

In ideal circumstances candidates for a co-ordinating role should possess the majority of the above skills and proven experience in managing a service of this type. Unfortunately, because of the novelty of this approach (at least in cardiac terms), such individuals are probably few and far between.

The training programme

All clinicians need to continually update their knowledge base and clinical skills. Moreover, it is important to provide a consistent level of care across the service. Before any of the appointed specialist nurses begin to recruit and assume responsibility for patients it is important – regardless of their expertise – that they all undergo a comprehensive training programme. In Glasgow, for example, all appointed specialist heart failure nurses undertake a comprehensive 4-week induction programme. Training programmes should incorporate the following topics:

- *The health-care system:*
  - how the various components of health care system are linked at an operational level
  - the role and cost of hospital-based health care
  - the role and cost of community-based health care
  - referring patients to other health-care professionals
  - co-ordinating health-care.

- *The heart failure patient:*
  - the pathophysiology of heart failure
  - identifying eligible patients
  - assessing the patient with heart failure
  - the "gold standard" pharmacological treatment of heart failure and the application of medical guidelines to optimise such treatment
  - non-pharmacological management of heart failure and applying nursing guidelines to optimise such therapy.

- *Record-keeping and auditing:*
  - data validity and reliability
  - word processing and database management

- report writing

- *Administrative issues:*
  - sick leave
  - complaints

- *Miscellaneous issues:*
  - medicolegal issues
  - security
  - professional development.

The training programme should also incorporate a large component of practical exposure to the day-to-day roles of the various health-care professionals who are commonly involved in the management of the heart failure patient (for example, hospital-based staff, general practitioner or primary care physician, dietitian and pharmacist). Visits to the homes of eligible heart failure patients are also required to fine-tune assessment skills and to ensure that protocols and guidelines can be properly and safely applied.

Step 9: Miscellaneous considerations

Creating or applying pre-existing guidelines and protocols

Whilst we have described a number of protocols describing the recruitment of patients and the interaction between the specialist nurse and the hospital and community-based health-care professionals, it is also important to create clear guidelines for the pharmacological and non-pharmacological management of the patient by the specialist nurse. The former is especially important if the specialist nurse is empowered to initiate and adjust pharmacotherapy. However, even if not so empowered, the nurse should be in a position to evaluate the effectiveness of prescribed therapy and initiate changes indirectly if required. Appendix I is an example of a comprehensive protocol for implementing and managing an appropriate pharmacological regimen for the management of chronic heart failure based on the Scottish Intercollegiate Guidelines Network (SIGN) guidelines.[4] Appendix II summarises the important components of non-pharmacological management of chronic heart failure.

Use of interpreters

The interaction between patients with heart failure, their treatment, and the health-care system in which they are managed, is a complex one. The probability of misunderstanding and mistakes damaging health outcomes is therefore high, particularly for individuals who do not speak the predominant language used within the health-care system. Dealing with such individuals is difficult and it should come as no surprise that with one major exception, the studies described in Chapter 3 either implicitly or explicitly excluded patients who did not speak the primary language of that region.

However, a service should be as inclusive as possible. In order to prepare for dealing with such patients, it is important that the training of the specialist nurses should include components of education that enhance cultural awareness and the appropriate use of interpreters (for example, when it is best to use a qualified interpreter rather than a family member). If it is anticipated that numerous patients will require interpreting services, then this should be included in the budget and formal links made to ensure rapid consultation when required.

Developing a patient information booklet

Older heart failure patients often have difficulty in remembering the details of their condition and their treatment – especially when their pharmacological regimen is being adjusted on a continuous basis. Health-care professionals also have difficulty in tracking the progress of the heart failure patient and appreciate a concise but accurate summary of both patient and treatment. A good way of facilitating patients' understanding of their condition and treatment and health-care professionals' management of the heart failure is to provide patients with an information booklet that is both educational and a record of their progress and treatment.

There are many different information booklets for heart failure patients, indicative of the many views on this subject. Rather than prescribing one particular format or booklet, we recommend a careful consideration of the "local" needs of the patients, the health-care professionals, and the health-care system itself (for example, regulatory and confidentiality requirements).

When developing a patient information and record booklet – whether adapting a pre-existing booklet or compiling a completely new one – there are a number of questions to consider:

- Who is the booklet primarily for? Is it for the patient, the health-care professional, or both? If designed simply to provide information about heart failure, the booklet will be solely directed at the patient. If it is also used to record the patient's treatment and progress then it will need to satisfy those health-care professionals who use it most.
- If the booklet is directed at the patient, has it been developed in collaboration with a typical group of heart failure patients who have advised on both content and language? If not, then it is likely to be too complex and also to concentrate on what the health-care professional thinks is important (for example, the pathophysiology of heart failure), not what the patient thinks is important (for example, how to cope with diuresis).

- If the booklet is to be used by health-care professionals, has the recording process and information been checked for accuracy, and the rule of absolute necessity, confidentiality, and practicality?
- Has it been approved by a person experienced in the graphic design and content of information booklets?

The following are some components that must be included in a heart failure booklet.

Records

Health-care professionals who have infrequent contact with the heart failure patient (for example, emergency service staff) appreciate up-to-date information concerning the patient's recent history and treatment. The records section should include:

- patient details
- contact details for the heart failure nurse, general practitioner, and ambulance and hospital services.
- baseline measurements relevant to the patient's condition (for example, degree of left ventricular systolic dysfunction)
- record of all appointments with the specialist nurse, cardiologist, and general practitioner
- current pharmacotherapy and any recent changes to the regimen
- a weight recording section
- an investigation recording section (for example, relating to electrolyte and renal function status).

Educational material

This should be easy to understand and provide the key points for each section. Patients or their families should be able to pick up the booklet and find what they want to know almost immediately. Topics should include:

- why is the heart so important?
- what is heart failure? (a drawing is often helpful)
- how do I know if I have heart failure?
- how does the doctor know if I have heart failure?
- how can I improve my health?
- exercising
- conserving energy
- managing fluid intake
- managing a "low-salt" diet
- managing medications (including sections on each major class of agent used in heart failure and a section on issues relating to treatment compliance)

- when to contact the heart failure nurse, doctor, or ambulance
- miscellaneous subjects such as smoking, managing angina, and alcohol intake
- a summary of key points.

Depending on the general purpose and content of the booklet, it may be sized either to sit on the patient's table at home as a reference work, or to fit in a pocket so patients can easily take it with them to a clinic or the hospital. If possible, the booklet should be constructed in a way that allows the content to be personalised (for example, removing the section on angiotensin-converting enzyme inhibitors if the patient is intolerant of this class of agent) so as to minimise the risk of "information overload".

Equipment

Many patients cannot afford simple items such as scales for weighing and measuring jugs to monitor their fluid status. If possible these items should be provided on loan, and their cost should be considered when budgeting for the service.

Equipment likely to be required by the specialist nurse includes:

- a computer with advanced word processing and data management capabilities
- a mobile telephone
- facsimile and answering machine
- a car (if home visits are required)
- a fully equipped clinic (if clinic visits are required)
- a sphygmomanometer and stethoscope
- venepuncture equipment with appropriate collection tubes.

All of these items, and the office space required, should be considered when costing this type of service.

Security

If specialist nurses are required to perform home visits, their safety is an important consideration. This entails reliable documentation of their visiting schedule and the availability of a personal alarm system – or at least an alert button on their mobile telephone – to seek emergency assistance.

Budgeting and resources

In any intervention of this type, there are many costs that remain hidden until the service becomes fully operational. Contrary to popular belief, it is not a simple matter of employing a specialist nurse and watching the health benefits flow thereafter. The following is a short list of the sort of costs that need to be accounted for when establishing this type of service:

- the specialist nurses (with coverage of sickness and annual leave)
- office and/or clinic space and equipment
- transport (for example, supplying a car and ongoing travel costs)
- communication (for example, telephone, paperwork and computing)
- monitoring equipment (for example, weighing machines and venepuncture equipment)
- additional investigations (for example, electrolyte and renal function tests)
- referral costs (for example, dietitian, social worker and pharmacist)
- record-keeping (for example, computer equipment)
- auditing
- patient booklets
- training costs (for example, a 4-week induction programme and ongoing educational activities).

Step 10: Undertake a final review of the service before formally recruiting patients

Introducing this type of intervention as a formal service is not easy without staff who are experienced in implementing and budgeting for new health-care services. Clearly there needs to be sufficient funding to provide the specialist nurses with both equipment and time to develop and implement effective protocols. With or without sufficient funding, however, the service will undoubtedly fail without the support of key personnel – ideally leading cardiologists, general practitioners or primary care physicians, and nurses for that particular region.

Prior to patient recruitment we would suggest a final review of the service development process to ensure that the following have been established, or at least considered:

- precise and realistic aims and objectives for the service
- close links with both the hospital and the community-based health-care services
- concise and realistic inclusion criteria for patients eligible to receive the service
- precise protocols for the identification and recruitment of hospitalised heart failure patients
- precise protocols for the careof the patient immediately after discharge (including the co-ordination of health care and the management of pharmacological and non-pharmacological treatment strategies)

- precise protocols for the longer-term management of the patient according to their risk of rehospitalisation and overall health-care needs
- comprehensive and independent auditing procedures
- a comprehensive list of infrastructure and equipment needs, ensuring that all items and service requirements are carefully accounted for
- a staff of specialist nurses recruited using strict selection criteria, who are adequately paid and are subject to a rigorous and comprehensive training programme
- an introduction period for the service allowing enough time for protocols to be tested properly and any teething problems to be adequately addressed.

To facilitate future developments of this kind in other regions and countries, it would be extremely useful for a "blueprint" of the developed service to be available for interested parties to obtain and consider.

Conclusion

Given sufficient funding and support, the recruitment of effective specialist nurses, and the application of carefully constructed protocols that ensure individualised health care, there is every likelihood that this type of service will improve health outcomes in patients unfortunate enough to be hospitalised with chronic heart failure. Unfortunately, given the complex nature of this type of intervention and the variations in health care inherent to each country there is no simple "prescription" for constructing a service. In this book, however, we have attempted to provide the most contemporary evidence supporting this kind of innovative approach to the management of heart failure and a preliminary "blueprint" for establishing a formal programme. We hope that the expertise required to develop and implement these programs will rapidly become more widespread, and that heart failure patients will enjoy more individualised and attentive care as a result.

References

1   Ekman I, Andersson B, Ehnfors M, Matejka B, Persson B, Fagerberg B. Feasability of a nurse-monitored, outpatient-care programme for elderly patients with moderate-to-severe, chronic heart failure. *Eur Heart J* 1998; **19**: 1254–60.
2   Folstein M, Folstein S, McHugh P. Mini-Mental State. A practical method for grading the cognitive state of patients for the clinician. *J Psychiatr Res* 1975; **12**: 189–98.
3   Weinberger M, Oddone EZ, Henderson WG. Does increased access to primary care reduce hospital readmissions? *N Engl J Med* 1996; **334**: 1441–7.
4   Scottish Intercollegiate Guidelines Network Scottish Cancer Therapy Network. *Diagnosis and treatment of heart failure due to left ventricular systolic dysfunction.* Edinburgh: Royal College of Physicians, 1999.

Appendix I: Guidelines for the pharmacological management of chronic heart failure

JOHN J V McMURRAY, LYNDA BLUE, SIMON STEWART

It is important to note that the following guidelines for the optimal pharmacological management of heart failure are an *example* only and that each service should create its own carefully constructed guidelines, taking into consideration the type of health care already provided and all medicolegal considerations.

The pharmacological management of chronic heart failure

Optimising the pharmacological treatment of chronic heart failure is one of the key components of specialist nurse-led interventions. For various reasons, many patients are receiving less than optimal pharmacological therapy at the time of their hospital discharge. Moreover, the dynamic and fluctuating nature of this syndrome means that the pharmacological regimen needs to be continually evaluated and adjusted.

The following description of the optimal pharmacotherapy for chronic heart failure is based on the Scottish Intercollegiate Guidelines Network (SIGN) guidelines for the management of heart failure secondary to left ventricular systolic dysfunction, prepared by a multidisciplinary working group chaired by Professor John McMurray from the Clinical Research Initiative in Heart Failure at the University of Glasgow, Scotland and endorsed by the NSF for England.[1]

"Gold standard" pharmacotherapy for chronic heart failure

In the absence of specific contraindications, all patients with heart failure due to left ventricular systolic dysfunction should be considered for treatment with an *angiotensin-converting enzyme (ACE) inhibitor*.

Patients with signs of sodium and water retention (peripheral oedema, pulmonary oedema, or an elevated jugular venous pressure), should also receive *diuretic therapy*.

The following patients should be considered for treatment with *digoxin*:

- all patients with heart failure and atrial fibrillation who need control of the ventricular rate, ß-blockers are, however, first choice therapy for this indication
- patients with moderately severe or severely symptomatic (New York Heart Association class III or IV) heart failure who remain symptomatic despite diuretic and ACE inhibitor therapy, have had more than one hospital admission for heart failure, and have very poor left ventricular systolic function or persisting cardiomegaly (a cardiothoracic ratio above 0.55).

Patients already treated with diuretics and/or digoxin and an ACE inhibitor, who are clinically stable and in NYHA classes I, II, or III, should be considered for treatment with a *ß-blocker*. Such patients should be under the careful supervision of a specialist.

Patients already treated with diuretics, an ACE inhibitor and/or digoxin who are in NYHA classes III or IV, should be considered for treatment with low-dose (25 mg orally, once daily) *spironolactone*. Careful monitoring of blood chemistry is mandatory.

Patients truly intolerant of an ACE inhibitor should be considered for treatment with *spironolactone*, *digoxin*, the combination of *hydralazine* and *isosorbide nitrate*, or an *angiotensin-II receptor antagonist*.

Patients with heart failure caused by coronary artery disease should be treated with an *HMG-CoA reductase inhibitor*.

Applying the guidelines

The following guidelines are to be used under the supervision of the patient's general practitioner and the responsible cardiologist for the service in each region. They include detailed protocols for the use of the evidence based treatments recommended by SIGN for patients with chronic heart failure caused by left ventricular systolic dysfunction.[1] Certain treatments must be discussed with the patient's general practitioner (ACE inhibitors, spironolactone, digoxin) or the contact cardiologist (ß-blocker) before initiation. The general practitioner may ask the specialist nurse to act as an intermediary and seek advice about medication from the responsible cardiologist. Any treatment initiation or dosage change must be communicated to all relevant parties (general practitioner, hospital personnel involved in continuing care) and recorded in the specific case records.

Angiotensin-converting enzyme inhibitor

Commencing therapy

Before starting an ACE inhibitor please consult the patient's general practitioner. Captopril, enalapril (trandolapril 4 mg once daily) are the preferred ACE inhibitors in this guideline and all patients should, if at all possible, be prescribed this class of agent. The target dose of captopril is three times daily, for enalapril it is 10–20 mg twice daily. Ramipril 10 mg once daily and lisinopril 30 mg once daily are equally acceptable alternatives. Every effort should be made to achieve the target dose (or as far as tolerated).

In the absence of severe asymptomatic hypotension (systolic blood pressure < 90 mmHg), symptomatic hypotension or significant renal impairment (serum creatinine ≥ 200 µmol/l and or urea ≥ 15 mmol/l), the dose of ACE inhibitor can be increased. If, however, any of these contraindications are present in a patient receiving a suboptimal dose of ACE inhibitor, seek medical advice. In the absence of a contraindication, increase the dose of enalapril in 2.5 mg increments and the dose of captopril in 12.5 mg increments (for example, enalapril 2.5 mgd, 5 mgd, 10 mg twice daily etc.). There should be at least 1 week between dose increments. Before the next dose increment contraindications should be checked for and, if present, medical advice should be sought. Blood pressure and blood chemistry must therefore be checked within 1 week of a dose increment and before the next dose increment.

Potential problems

Cough, hypoperfusion (cerebral and renal) and angio-oedema are the major adverse effects associated with ACE inhibitor therapy. If a patient has a genuinely troublesome cough clearly related to the ACE inhibitor an angiotensin-II receptor antagonist should be substituted – *please seek medical advice.*

Cerebral hypoperfusion presents as dizziness, blackouts, lightheadedness, etc. Very often this can be resolved by reducing concomitant medications (i.e. diuretics and, especially nitrates and calcium channel blockers). If this problem arises please seek medical advice. It is important to note that patients taking an ACE inhibitor may have a low blood pressure and no symptoms (asymptomatic hypotension). This finding does not necessitate any action unless there is renal hypoperfusion. Renal hypoperfusion leads to an increase in serum levels of urea, creatinine, and often also potassium. Small increases in urea, creatinine, and potassium are common and acceptable consequences of using an ACE inhibitor. If potassium levels exceed 5.5 mmol/l the ACE inhibitor must be stopped immediately, at least temporarily, *and medical advice should be sought.* If the urea level increases to 20 mmol/l or more (or by more than 10 mmol/l) or creatinine to 300 μmol/l or more (or by more than 100 μmol/l) the ACE inhibitor should again be stopped immediately. Very often deteriorating renal function is due to overdiuresis and dehydration (for example, due to diarrhoea and vomiting) or other concomitant medication (especially non-steroidal anti-inflammatory agents and potassium-sparing diuretics). *Medical advice should be sought* with respect to adjustment or discontinuation of these concomitant treatments. Less serious increases (i.e. urea 5–10 mmol/l or creatinine 50–100 μmol/l) should be monitored very closely. Blood chemistry should be checked every second day and *medical advice should be sought.*

Small changes in serum concentrations of urea (< 5 mmol/l) and creatinine (< 50 μmol/l) can be ignored provided these changes are stable (i.e. show no progression between two blood tests at least 2 weeks apart).

Loop diuretics

Commencing therapy

The majority of patients with heart failure are prescribed a loop diuretic. On reviewing the patient, determine whether the diuretic agent has been prescribed in a daily dose sufficient to achieve "dry" weight (the goal of treatment). In other words, is the patient oedema-free and is the jugular venous pressure (JVP) normal? Also determine whether patients are aware that their diuretic dose need not be constant (for example, postponement of the morning dose to ensure a comfortable shopping trip or travel is perfectly acceptable).

Dose adjustments

The dose of diuretic should be increased if the patient shows a sustained (≥ 3 days) and significant (≥ 0.5 kg) increase in weight above "dry" weight, especially if this is accompanied by an increase in peripheral oedema, JVP, or symptoms of breathlessness. The patient's diuretic dose should be increased, initially for 3 days; the dose increment should be maintained and medical advice sought if dry weight is not regained by the end of 3 days of increased therapy. If the patient is taking 40 mg of frusemide (bumetanide equivalent = 1 mg) once daily, the dose should be increased to 80 mg once daily. If the patient is taking 80 mg once daily the dose should be increased to 80 mg once (morning) and 40 mg once (lunchtime) daily. If the patient is taking 80 mg and 40 mg once daily the dose should be increased to 80 mg twice daily. If the patient is taking 80 mg frusemide twice daily or more *medical advice should be sought* before increasing the dose of diuretic. Decreasing the diuretic dose should only be done cautiously and the patient should be contacted 48 hours later to assess the response to the dose reduction. The dose should be reduced from the usual maintenance dose only if there are signs of volume depletion and hypoperfusion. There should, therefore, be evidence of significant weight loss from dry weight ($\geq$ 1 kg), a rising concentration of blood urea ($\geq$ 5 mmol/l or $\geq$ 25%) and/or symptoms of dizziness (for example, postural hypotension) or feeling "dried out". The dose of diuretic should *not* be reduced if there is peripheral oedema, or if the JVP is elevated to 7 cm or more from the sternal angle. If the patient has a rising blood urea level, falling weight and/or symptoms of dizziness or dehydration, but peripheral oedema – *please seek medical advice*. Overall, the dose of diuretic should not be decreased to below 40 mg of frusemide (or equivalent) without seeking medical advice. *If in doubt seek medical advice*. Dose reduction of frusemide should be carried out in 40 mg decrements (the reverse of the up-titration schedule outlined above). If the patient is taking more than 80 mg frusemide twice daily *seek medical advice* before changing the dose.

Potential problems

Unfortunately, taking a loop diuretic (frusemide or bumetanide) after 1600–1800 hours can lead to nocturia. Moreover, too great a diuresis can cause dizziness, lightheadedness, fatigue (or a "washed-out" feeling), and uraemia. This can be a particular problem if the patient becomes dehydrated for another reason (diarrhoea, vomiting, hot weather, poor fluid intake); gout can also occur. Usually the patient will show a significant ($\geq$ 1 kg) and sustained decrease in weight below dry weight. The patient's JVP may not be visible at 45°.

Thiazide diuretics and metolazone

Thiazides and related diuretics may be used as an *alternative* to loop diuretics in patients with less severe heart failure or in *addition* to loop diuretics in patients with very severe heart failure. Unlike loop diuretics, thiazides and metolazone are long-acting, and adjustment of the timing of the dose is not advantageous as for loop diuretics. Otherwise the principles of use, monitoring, and potential problems are similar to those of loop diuretics. The combination of a thiazide or metolazone, and a loop diuretic must be used with extreme caution and *only after careful medical consultation*. Close biochemical monitoring of such combination therapy is mandatory. Thiazides and metolazone can also cause hyponatraemia, in addition to the other biochemical problems discussed under loop diuretics. If the serum sodium concentration falls below 133 mmol/l *medical advice should be sought immediately*.

Spironolactone

Commencing therapy

Spironolactone treatment should only be started after discussion with the patient's general practitioner. Patients who remain symptomatic on less than ordinary activity (those in NYHA class III or IV despite treatment with a diuretic), an ACE inhibitor and, where indicated, a ß-blocker, should be considered for treatment with spironolactone. Patients with persisting signs of sodium and water retention (for example, peripheral oedema) may be particularly suitable for this treatment.

Before commencing therapy, check the patient's baseline blood chemistry (see potential problems below). The starting dose of spironolactone is 25 mg once daily (a lower dose may be used where there is concern – see cautions above). Check the patient's blood chemistry after 1 week, 2 weeks, and 4 weeks of treatment. Further checks of blood chemistry should be made every 4 weeks for 3 months, then every 3 months for 1 year, and every 6 months thereafter. Treatment should be stopped and *medical advice sought* as outlined below.

Potential problems

The patient may become sodium- and water-depleted and hypovolaemic on spironolactone, necessitating a reduction in the dose of potassium-losing diuretic (for example, frusemide) or discontinuation of the spironolactone. This can be expected if the patient complains of postural dizziness or lightheadedness, there is sustained hypotension, a significant and sustained weight loss ($\geq$ 1 kg, sustained over more than a week), the presence of a comorbid condition associated with sodium and water depletion (for example, diarrhoea and vomiting – *if this occurs, stop spironolactone immediately*) or if the patient has not been drinking fluids or has been in a hot climate and perspiring excessively.

Discontinue spironolactone and *seek advice from the senior cardiologist* should the patient experience *any* of the following *at any time*:

- an increase in serum creatinine concentration to 250 µmol/l or more, or by 25% or more from baseline (for example, from 80 µmol/l to 100 µmol/l).
- an increase in serum urea concentration to 18 mmol/l or more, or by 50% or more from baseline, for example, from 8 mmol/l to 12 mmol/l.
- an increase in serum potassium concentration to 5.5 mmol/l or more.
- diarrhoea or vomiting (or any other cause of sodium and water loss).

Digoxin

Commencing therapy

Digoxin seems to provide symptomatic benefit to patients with chronic heart failure – even if they are in sinus rhythm. It also appears to reduce hospital admissions for heart failure, especially in those patients with severe heart failure as suggested by a very low left ventricular ejection fraction (LVEF) and cardiomegaly.

Dose adjustments

Most trials showing a benefit from digoxin treatment used a mean daily dose of 0.375 mg, though in a recent trial the average dose was 0.25 mg (given once daily). The dose used should be aimed at achieving a serum concentration within the therapeutic range (0.6–2.6 nmol/l). If a patient receiving digoxin does not have a therapeutic serum concentration and has a creatinine level of 200 μmol/l or more and urea level of 15 mmol/l or more, the dose should be increased by 0.0625 mg and the plasma concentration rechecked, 6 hours post-dose, in approximately 2 weeks. This process of up-titration should be repeated until a therapeutic concentration is achieved or a dose of 0.5 mg has been reached. *Seek medical advice* if a dose of 0.5 mg, but not a therapeutic concentration, has been reached.

Potential problems

If a patient has severely abnormal renal function (serum concentration of creatinine 200 μmol/l or more or urea 15 mmol/l or more) or has not been prescribed digoxin, *seek medical advice*. Digoxin toxicity can arise with any dose of digoxin but is more common when the therapeutic concentration is exceeded. Anorexia, nausea, vomiting, xanthopsia, bradycardia, and ventricular arrhythmias are the classically recognised effects of digoxin toxicity. In elderly patients the symptoms and signs of digoxin toxicity may be non-specific. These may include confusion (either new-onset or increasing), deteriorating mobility, and falls. Digoxin should be withheld, at least temporarily, if any of these occur, an urgent assessment of serum digoxin concentration should be made and *medical advice should be sought immediately*.

Plasma digoxin concentrations most commonly increase because of deteriorating renal function and because of drug interactions (amiodarone and erythromycin are two major culprits in this regard). Digoxin-induced arrhythmias (for example, *torsades de pointes*) are much more common in hypokalaemic patients. Close monitoring of blood chemistry is, therefore, the key to the safe use of digoxin, particularly where there is a change in drug therapy or instability (for example, a change in the dose of diuretic; initiation or increase in dose of ACE inhibitor; initiation of amiodarone or erythromycin; diarrhoea or vomiting, or any other upset that might affect renal function).

Beta-blockers

Commencing therapy

It has been demonstrated that certain ß-blockers reduce mortality (by about one-third) and hospital admissions (by about 20%) when added to full conventional heart failure therapy, including ACE inhibitor treatment. It should be noted that treatment must only be initiated and titrated under close supervision of an individual expert in the management of heart failure, usually a specialist hospital physician.

The above restrictions, of course, closely resemble those imposed during the initial introduction of ACE inhibitors. Many will remember monitoring patients in the hospital setting when initiating an ACE inhibitor. There is little doubt that, as the general experience of ß-blocker management in heart failure increases, the initiation and titration of such therapy will become less restricted.

Eligible patients are those with a confirmed diagnosis of chronic heart failure due to left ventricular systolic dysfunction, in NYHA class II or III, already receiving standard therapy (a diuretic, an ACE inhibitor, and possibly digoxin) and, importantly, those who are clinically stable – meaning patients who have had no adjustment in pharmacotherapy within 4 weeks and no hospitalisation within 2 months, a heart rate of 55 beats per minute or more and a systolic blood pressure of 90 mmHg or more and no contraindication to ß-blockade (for example, bradyarrhythmias or asthma). It is permissible to start ß-blockers in sicker, more unstable, patients but this decision should only be made by a hospital specialist at present and treatment initiated and titrated under the care of such a specialist.

Dose adjustments

Beta-blocker therapy must be initiated at the lowest dose and increased slowly. The titration intervals shown should be regarded as the *minimum* intervals, see Figure A1. After the first dose of treatment patients should ideally be observed for hypotension, bradycardia, or worsening heart failure for 2–3 hours (carvedilol) or approximately 4 hours (bisoprolol). Patients must be advised of possible adverse effects and to seek assistance from the specialist nurse should these occur. Before each dosage increase patients must be reviewed for adverse effects and signs of worsening heart failure.

Potential adverse effects

Adverse events during the initiation and up-titration of ß-blockers in heart failure are not uncommon and patients will often experience temporary deterioration of their heart failure symptoms. This is minimised

The following guidance reflects the current summaries of product characteristics (as of November 1999):

- observe indications and contraindications
- treatment must only be initiated and titrated "under the supervision of a hospital physician" (carvedilol) or "a physician experienced in the treatment of heart failure" (bisoprolol)
- therapy must be initiated in the hospital setting at the lowest dose (see below) and up-titrated *slowly* (see below) – the titration intervals shown should be regarded as the *minimum* intervals
- after the first dose of treatment patients must be observed for hypotension, bradycardia or worsening CHF for 2–3 hours (carvedilol) or approximately 4 hours (bisoprolol)
- patients must be advised of possible adverse effects and to seek assistance (according to local arrangements), should these occur before each dose up-titration patients must be reviewed for adverse effects and signs of worsening heart failure
- patients must also be observed for 2–3 hours after each dose up-titration of carvedilol
- patients must be advised of possible adverse effects and to seek assistance (according to local arrangements), should these occur.

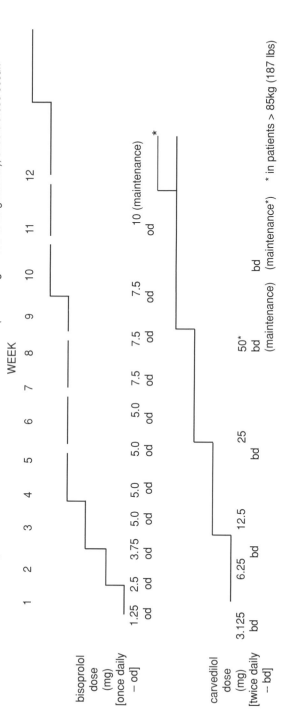

Figure A1 Titrating beta blocker therapy in CHF (metoprolol CR/XL, used in MERIT-HF, is not available in the UK)

by careful patient selection, use of a small initial dose of ß-blocker, and slow and cautious dose up-titration. Usually initial problems can be overcome by adjustment of the dose of concomitant medications and the majority of appropriate patients can be readily established on ß-blocker therapy. Generally, ß-blocker therapy should not be stopped suddenly, though this may be necessary if the patient develops a significant bradycardia or worsening of symptoms (including symptomatic hypotension).

It is helpful to advise patients that a ß-blocker is prescribed primarily with the objective of maintaining stability and preventing progression of heart failure in the longer term. No immediate symptomatic improvement is expected, and initially there may be some symptom worsening before improvement occurs. Patients may become more breathless or oedematous (or gain weight) due to a worsening of their heart failure. Usually this can be corrected by increasing the dose of diuretic (this may only be necessary on a temporary basis). Normally the patient should improve within 2–3 days. If the patient does not improve within 1 week consider decreasing (or stopping) the dose of ß-blocker. Wait 4 weeks before attempting further dose up-titration (or reintroduction) of ß-blocker therapy.

If the patient experiences symptomatic hypotension, consider overdiuresis and whether reduction in the dose of diuretic may improve matters. Also consider discontinuing other hypotensive drugs of no definite value in heart failure (for example, nitrates, calcium channel blockers, α-adrenoceptor blockers). The patient's dose of ACE inhibitor may also need to be decreased temporarily. If the problem is unresolved, decrease the dose of (or stop) the ß-blocker. Wait 4 weeks before attempting further dose up-titration (or reintroduction) of ß-blocker therapy.

If the systolic blood pressure falls to below 90 mmHg the patient's blood chemistry should be checked. Advice should be sought if the changes detailed above for diuretics and ACE inhibitors occur (usually the dose of ß-blocker should be reduced).

If the patient's heart rate falls below 55 beats per minute, reduce the dose to the previous dose level (for example, 10 mg to 5 mg of bisoprolol). If the symptoms are serious, consider stopping treatment immediately. Review within 1 week and reduce the dose further if the heart rate is still below 55/min. Review the medication regimen, and consider reducing or completely stopping other drugs that can slow sinoatrial and atrioventricular conduction (for example, digoxin, diltiazem, and amiodarone). If the patient's heart rate falls below 40 beats per minute stop the ß-blocker and arrange for a 12-lead electrocardiogram to be performed. *Referral to a cardiologist is advised*. This is because such a low heart rate may indicate that ß-blocker therapy has precipitated second- or third-degree atrioventricular block ("heart block") or sick sinus syndrome.

Blood chemistry monitoring

When a patient is referred to the service, *baseline* measurements of blood chemistry should be recorded (sodium, potassium, urea, creatinine). After any sustained (> 1 week) doubling of diuretic dose, blood chemistry must be rechecked within a week. Increases in urea and creatinine and increases or decreases in potassium levels are of concern. If the urea concentration increases to 20 mmol/l or more (or by more than 10 mmol/l) or the creatinine concentration increases to 300 μmol/l or more (or by more than 100 μmol/l) *immediate advice should be sought* (generally, in the absence of signs of salt and water retention, the dose of diuretic should be reduced). If the potassium concentration decreases to 3.5 mmol/l or below *immediate advice should be sought* (generally, in the absence of signs of salt and water retention, the dose of diuretics should be reduced; alternatively, the dose of ACE inhibitor can be increased or spironolactone added). If the potassium concentration increases to 5.5 mmol/l or above *immediate advice should be sought* (generally, in the absence of signs of salt and water retention, the dose of diuretic should be reduced; alternatively the dose of ACE inhibitor may need to be reduced, or spironolactone or non-steroidal anti-inflammatory drugs may need to be discontinued).

Reference

1   Scottish Intercollegiate Guidelines Network – Scottish Cancer Therapy Network. *Diagnosis and treatment of heart failure due to left ventricular systolic dysfunction.* Edinburgh: Royal College of Physicians, 1999.

Appendix II: Guidelines for the non-pharmacological management of chronic heart failure

SIMON STEWART, LYNDA BLUE

There are a number of strategies that can supplement and increase the effectiveness of the pharmacological treatment of heart failure. Their relative potency should not be underestimated: as witnessed by the fact that most trials of pharmacological agents require thousands of patients to prove efficacy, whilst trials of nurse-led strategies have typically recruited fewer than 300 patients. However, non-pharmacological strategies are undoubtedly effective when implemented concurrently and not singularly. We cannot, for example, identify which one of the strategies described below is most effective, or alternatively can be omitted with confidence from the repertoire of the specialist nurse.

The non-pharmacological management of chronic heart failure

Education and counselling

Patients and their family and carers where appropriate, should be made aware of the purpose, effects and potential adverse effects, of their pharmacological treatment, and if necessary receive additional information about heart failure itself. This can be achieved through a combination of educational strategies including personal counselling in the home, written materials, and referral to the patient's local pharmacist.

Facilitating treatment adherence

As non-adherence to treatment is common, it is safe to assume that the majority of patients are having difficulty with their pharmacological regimen

155

and would benefit from advice and support in this regard. The greater the number of individual doses and medications, the greater the probability of non-adherence. The use of a prescription box is commonly indicated, or it may be possible to increase adherence by introducing a more realistic dosing schedule that suits the patient's life-style. It is also possible to encourage family or carers to take a more active role in ensuring that medications are managed correctly. Patients who demonstrate a good understanding of their condition and its treatment can be easily taught to increase or decrease their diuretic regimen in response to weight changes and their symptomatic profile.

Daily weight monitoring

Where possible, determine the patient's ideal "dry" weight (when a patient who has had signs of fluid retention after diuretic treatment reaches a steady weight at which there are no further signs of fluid overload). Using this ideal weight as a goal, encourage patients to weigh themselves daily and record their weight in the chart provided (usually in the patient booklet). If the patient does not have a suitable set of scales, provide one (see Chapter 10). The patient should be advised that the best time for weighing is:

- every morning
- after going to toilet and
- before getting dressed and
- before breakfast.

Instruct patients (or family and carers where appropriate) that a steady weight gain over a number of days may indicate that they are retaining too much fluid. If this gain in weight is more than 1 kg (2 lb) they should contact the specialist nurse. Conversely, patients who lose a similar amount of weight over the same sort of period should also contact the nurse in case they experience overdiuresis.

Controlled salt intake

The majority of heart failure patients, particularly those with marked fluid retention, will benefit from a reduction in salt intake. These patients should be advised to avoid salt-rich foods and the addition of supplemental salt to food when cooking. Where appropriate, patients should be referred for specialist review and advice from a dietitian (for example, patients with excessive fluid retention).

Exercise

Wherever possible patients should be offered an individualised exercise programme with encouragement to continue exercise thereafter. Patients with concurrent conditions likely to complicate the introduction of an exercise programme (for example, chronic airways disease, arthritis, or diabetes) require more specialist advice from an exercise physiologist. An exercise programme is much more likely to be beneficial if the patient is receiving optimal therapy and is clinically stable.

Controlling alcohol intake

For patients with alcohol-induced cardiomyopathy, alcohol is absolutely contraindicated. For others with chronic heart failure, alcohol may be consumed in small quantities, for example, one or two units per day.

Smoking

A patient's willingness to stop smoking should be determined, so that assistance can be given to those willing to attempt quitting, and motivational intervention given to those who are unwilling or equivocal. Strategies for smoking cessation should be tailored for each individual. The appropriate use of *nicotine replacement therapy* should be discussed with patients wishing to stop smoking.

Weight control

For management of obesity, a programme involving small, stepped changes towards a more modest target will have greater success than one aiming directly for a large weight loss. Many patients gain benefit from a group effect. Nutritional counselling by a health professional skilled in weight management and behaviour change should be offered.

Cardiac cachexia

Cardiac cachexia is a serious condition and is usually present in those patients with severe, end-stage heart failure. Ideally, a physician working in co-operation with a dietician should manage cachexia. Strategies may include altering meal size and frequency, and energy and vitamin supplementation of the patient's oral intake. The muscle wasting associated with cardiac cachexia also exacerbates exercise intolerance and enhances the sense of fatigue and dyspnoea. Every effort should be made to ensure adequate nutrition for these patients.

Psychological support

Although there is a paucity of data to support the use of psychological interventions for patients with heart failure, there is little doubt that it is both valuable and greatly appreciated. Depression, anxiety, and fear are common among those with heart failure.

While there are no specific recommendations to make about providing psychological support, it is important to determine whether the patient (or their immediate family or carers) are suffering from any form of psychological distress, and if so to arrange for more formal assessment and treatment. Otherwise, it is imperative that the specialist nurse allows time for the patient to discuss problems and issues of concern.

Immunisation

All patients with chronic heart failure should be advised to ask their general practitioner for an annual influenza immunisation and a single pneumoccocal immunisation.

Index